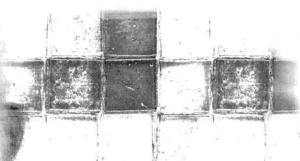

firewalkers

madness, beauty & mystery

RADICALLY RETHINKING MENTAL ILLNESS

Emotional turbulence

Spiritual breakthroughs

Visionary meltdowns

Altered states

Ecstatic visions

Crazy blessings

& Mad gifts

Firewalkers was created by people who have experienced extreme mental states (commonly labeled "mental illness")

FIREWALKERS STORYTELLERS

Myra Anderson

Carla Beck

Debra Knighton

Joni Michelle

Michelle Sese-Khalid

Lauren Spiro

Tracy D. Stuart

FIREWALKERS EDITORIAL TEAM

Cassandra Nudel
Firewalkers Creator & Photographer

Ann Benner
Program Leadership & Administrator

Malaina Poore
Firewalkers Coordinator

Bev Ball

Debra Knighton

Yolande Long

Ken Moore

Brian Parrish

Cynthia Power

Mitzi Ware

This book was created by **VOCAL**, a non-profit mental health community, support network, social change movement, and self-help education program in Virginia. Learn more about VOCAL and the Firewalkers project in the back of this book or visit us at <u>www.thefirebook.org</u>.

Underground Advertising collaborated in creating art direction, creative strategy, book design, and outreach materials for this project. <u>www.undergroundads.com</u>.

Deepest gratitude to Carol McLaughlin for superb transcription; Tracy Stuart & Arlene Jordan for editing gifts; Heather Peck for collaboration and adventure; Wendy MacNaughton for creative strategy; John Givens for art direction and book design; Heath Wickline for communications training and coordination; Lindsay Meisel for invaluable editing/organizing; Darlene Vandegrift for insight and illumination; and our wonderful colleagues John Otenasek & Bonnie Neighbour. Cover painting by Matt Manley. <u>www.mattmanley.com</u>, cover design by John Givens.

What is to give light
must endure burning.

–Viktor Frankl

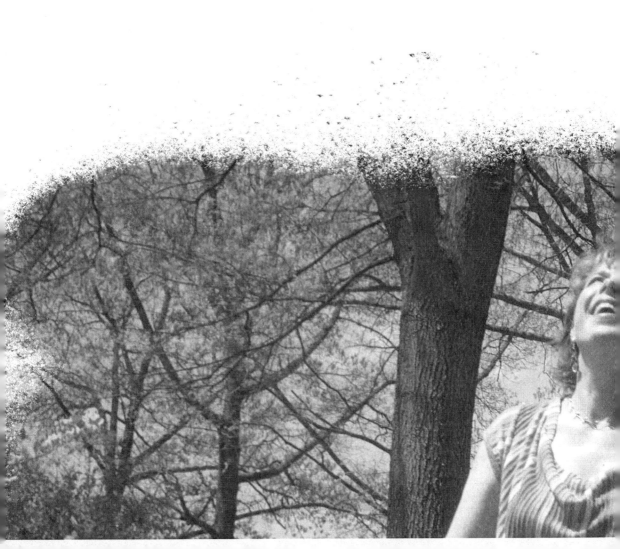

Contents

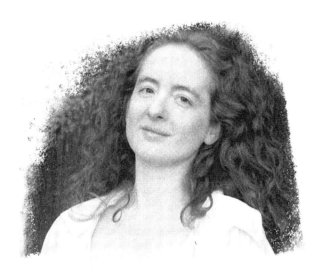

Illumination through Burning

Editor's Preface ~ Cassandra Nudel

The Sacred Quest

When we set out to create *Firewalkers*, we wanted people to know a mental health diagnosis is not a death sentence. It's not the end of the line or the last thing that will ever happen in your life. It's a strange and unexpected journey that most of us never asked for or ever wanted. But after walking through the fire, it has brought us somewhere. And for some of us, we would not go back. Even if we could.

We set out on a quest. We were looking for a different kind of story – something transcendent and profound and ecstatic and unearthing. My hope was to find people who not only said, "I survived mental illness" or, "I am recovering from mental illness" or even, "I am now recovered from mental illness," but people who went beyond that to say:

> *This was my life calling. My experiences with mental health crisis or the mental health system turned me into that person I was meant to be. This is my story, the dark journey I traveled, and this is where I arrived. How I found myself. How I discovered who I was meant to be in the world. How I traveled the hot coals and got burned and came through – not unscathed, but somewhat scathed and somewhat tired and somewhat lost and also somewhat open and somewhat full of wonder and somewhat full of hope. That is what mental illness was for me: It's the path I was meant to go down.*

We looked across our state for seven people who have experienced extreme states of consciousness. Altered states. Ecstatic visions. Spiritual breakdowns and spiritual breakthroughs. What our society labels "mental illness." We looked for people who have lived deeply through this experience, and through this experience have learned things they never expected to learn and become people they never expected to be. People who have faced madness, fire, creativity, the dark night of the soul, and the rich world beneath the surface, and now have a story to tell.

The Mustard Seed of Hope

Our editorial team was spectacular. Magical. The best team I have ever found or has ever found me. *Firewalkers* was a journey for us all. We collected stories from 34 people, interviewed 15 finalists, selected 7 for the book. We conducted 21 interviews, transcribed 400 pages, collected several hundred more pages of writing, traveled to people's homes, took 2,000 photographs, put it all in the cauldron, and hoped that somehow a book would come out. I didn't know when I started what it would take to get to the end of this. Thankfully, or I might never have started.

The thing I remember most vividly from our selection committee was calling Michelle and how when we asked her about recovery she spoke of "the mustard seed of hope." She had sent us her written story earlier, and it was so dark and mysterious and mystical and shattering in a way. Then we got on the phone with her and her voice was just filled with light and beauty and radiance. For a minute, I panicked and thought I had called the wrong person. That evening I got an email from someone else on the selection committee, "I am still under the illusion that we spoke with an angel."

Firewalkers is a mix and tumble. As you read the stories, you'll find there are people who were helped by medication and people who were harmed by it. People who were supported by hospitalization and people who were traumatized by it. People who believe mental illness is a medical disorder and people who believe mental illness does not exist.

We wanted to include it all, and we know we did not include it all. The most immediate and obvious piece missing is more stories from men. The vast majority of people who contacted us to be in the book were women. We wrestled with it and, in the end, chose to follow the seven stories where our hearts were most drawn. There are many wonderful people and many amazing stories that are not here. Perhaps another book. Another day.

Fire Dreams

The idea that mental illness can be a profound spiritual calling is not a concept I expect everyone to agree with. I know there will be a lot of people who read this book and don't resonate with this idea at all. But for some people it could be the defining moment. At least it was for me.

What I want is for us to be a song of hope. When I first started having mental and physical health collapse, my world was just went dark. Everything was just awash in despair. There was no sense around me that what I was going through could be a profound life change, a kind of spiritual awakening that could change me fundamentally. I had no knowing that that was possible.

In the wake of the shooting tragedy at Virginia Tech, many of us have noticed a change in the climate and culture of our state. The mental health laws have changed to be more restrictive and oppressive, and the media reports have spread fear, like fire, about people who have been diagnosed with mental illness and how violent and dangerous we may be. In creating *Firewalkers*, we want to give a different way of viewing mental illness and create a deeper understanding of what it means and what is possible.

We want *Firewalkers* to be different than what is already out there. There is already a lot of writing about stories of people with mental illness – but we rarely hear the story of the deep growth and transformation that can come through this journey. The ways our lives change in ways we never imagined. The people we become that we never thought we could be. The way after we walk through the fire, and everything burns away from us, our lives become different and – for some of us – deeper, richer, and strangely more powerful.

Mental health crisis can be hard. It can be hell. It can be barely survivable or unsurvivable. It can be the one great challenge of your life.

But it can also be something else.
An unearthing. An opening place. A path of discovery.
An illumination through burning.

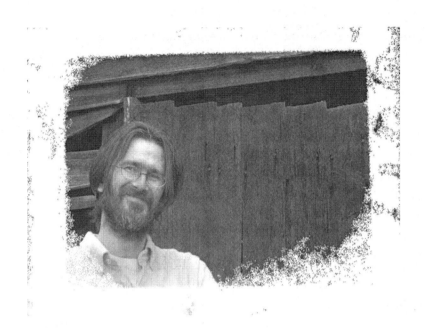

Stirring the Coals

An Introduction ~ Brian Parrish

This is a story about firewalkers. About people who walk through fire.

What is it, to go through this firewalk of mental illness? By its very nature, this journey is not easy, and it is not something most of us would do willingly. A turning point is passed. Many of us have no idea what is happening to us, but through trial and error, and sometimes without any recognizable signposts, we start to grow and change. It can seem like operating in the dark, but over time, you begin to shift and see new surroundings. The burning away of some things gives rise to others, and sometimes we can discover long hidden sensitivities, talents, and callings.

Often your greatest weakness is also where you find your greatest strength. When it comes to mental health and mental illness, we're fairly aware of the negatives. There's a really thick book that will tell us all about the down side, for as long as we're willing to listen. But could it be that what we are diagnosing as mental illness is in fact a search for wholeness, a search for balance and meaning in a sometimes painful and irrational world? Could it be that people who have been labeled with mental illness also have specialized sensitivities and abilities that others don't develop?

In our culture people are labeled with schizophrenia. In some Native American traditions, these same people are seen as being in touch with the spirit world. A person whom we might diagnose as having a mental illness may instead be considered to be a healer: a shaman, a medicine man or woman. The obvious danger in getting in touch with the spirit world would be to fall out of touch with everyday reality. Swimming in the spirit world, you can swim out of reach from the shore. You can be pulled out of reach. But there might be an ability there — an ability to walk between the worlds; to be attuned to people's hidden wounds and hearts. There's something about being able to go to that other place that allows you to start to see the world in a symbolic or different way.

Madness and genius are not opposites.

Others are labeled as manic. It seems to me that when someone is manic there is this amazing ability to make quantum leaps of understanding, to make creative connections, to have these stupendous "aha" moments. Of course, once I get a good night's sleep, it might turn out that I can't understand what I meant while I was up there, and some of it doesn't even seem to be in English. And then I find the diamond in the rough—the brilliant new idea that just might transform the world. And sometimes, just sometimes, it was all worth it.

Some of us are told we have anxiety disorder and post traumatic stress syndrome. I know based on my own childhood and early life, that sometimes things happened that were dangerous and I had to learn to live with them when I couldn't avoid them. Some research shows that when people have so-called "anxiety disorders," part of what they're actually doing is picking up subtle information in their immediate environment. They're picking up data that others are simply not aware of, cues that danger is possibly present. Their nervous system is like a spider web. It's very sensitively attuned; spiders need to know when something is touching their web. For some of us, our nervous systems are highly sensitive to sudden noise or light or conflict. Our ability might be to sense hidden dangers that others might miss.

With obsessive compulsive disorder, if our only information were gathered from movies and television, we'd think it was all about checking and rechecking the lock, lining up pencils in straight lines, or not walking on the cracks in sidewalks. It has been my observation that when these same people are on a project of researching information or combing through data or rearranging someone's living room, they can have amazing abilities in organizing and analyzing complex material.

In the end, what a society labels to be "mental illness" may be no more than a judgment, from a particular time and perspective, tinged with the preconceptions, needs, and fears of the culture doing the judging. For example, it wasn't until 1973 that sexual orientation disturbance (homosexuality) was retired from the *The Diagnostic and Statistical Manual of Mental Disorders*.

If we are to be successful in reclaiming our personal transformative experiences, it falls to us to redefine the terms. We can use the tools of language to reflect this. Of course, everyone's journey will be different, and so will the wording. To begin with, I think the term "mental" is misleading, for many experience their symptoms throughout their body. For some, the experience is intensely spiritual. Others may feel the experience deeply in their emotions. In the spirit of diversity and exploration, I offer the following to begin the dialogue: spiritual emergency, emotional turbulence, body-mind meltdown. Please feel free to mix and match.

Western medicine treats the symptoms without looking at the underlying imbalance. It misses the forest for the trees. It sees mental health symptoms as a problem to be stamped out, and doesn't see the holistic picture: There is something off-balance that needs to be gently righted, not medicated out of existence. If you think of one piece of a person as having to be medicated out of existence, you may be blunting them of their other gifts.

Madness and genius are not opposites. There is a circle, and madness and genius touch. Many great artists struggle with madness. Musicians can go on journeys out of their bodies and bring back amazing songs. Some painters are able to see visions of beauty that we would never lay eyes upon, were it not for their gifts and willingness to share. Writers with some of the most powerful voices often seem driven by tumultuous inner forces. It is no surprise to me, then, that artists can be at risk for addictions to drugs and alcohol, which also puts them out of their bodies. Without their inner voice and vision, all of our lives would be so much grayer.

Now, it's a common understanding that you can't give one thing up without replacing it with another. If you want to give up cigarettes, you'll want to put something in their place. Nature abhors a vacuum. So, if we say stigma about mental illness is bad and we want to get rid of it, then I ask: what are we replacing it with? If we are trying to change people's attitudes, what attitudes are we replacing them with? With *Firewalkers,* our goal is to look at the flip side and give people something different to consider.

Firewalkers is the story of seven people, ordinary people, who have walked through the fire. We hope their stories bring light to a new way of understanding the journey.

Seven Firewalkers

STORIES & INTERVIEWS

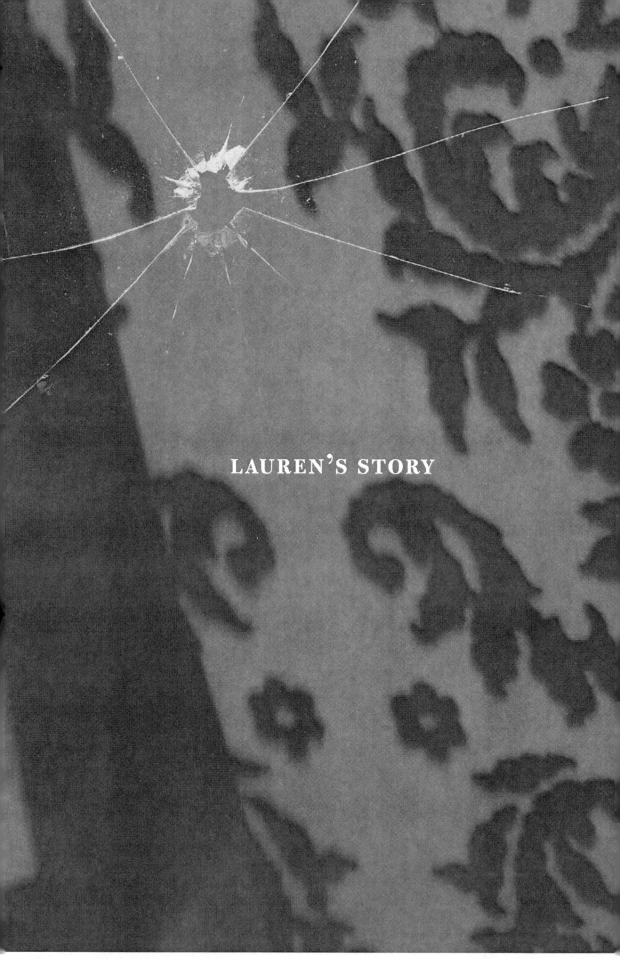

LAUREN'S STORY

I spent over 20 years believing that I had a mental illness,

that something was wrong with my brain.
I was told it was incurable and
I would spend the rest of my life
on psychiatric medication.

Now I've come to believe
that what I was told
was not true.

THE EXPERTS WERE WRONG.

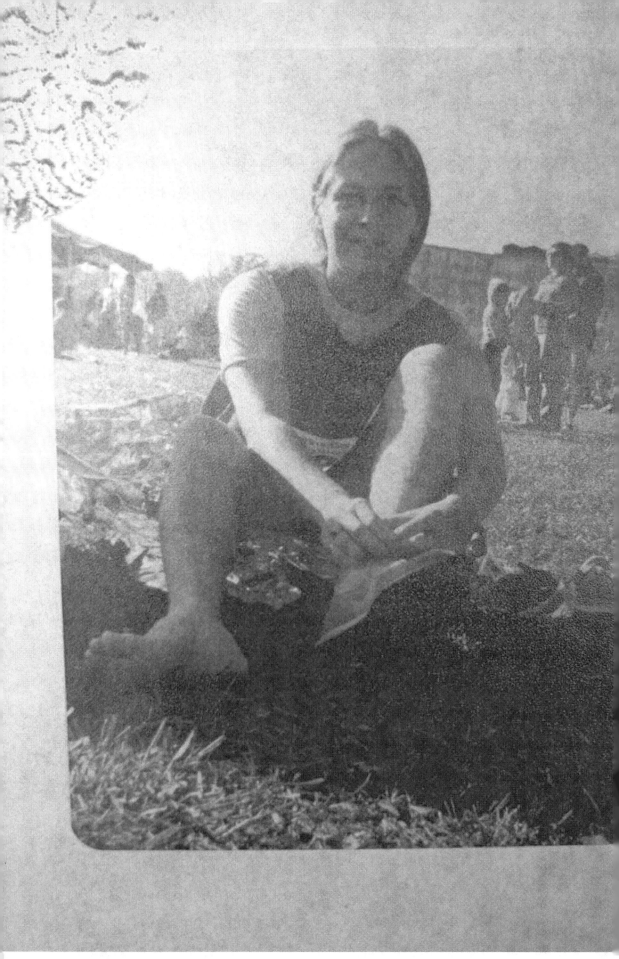

At the age of 16, I had what some would term a "break-down." I now call it a "breakthrough." Very quickly, and with almost no warning, my perception of myself was transformed. Suddenly, I felt I had a world-changing task, and I needed to talk to the President. It was so extraordinary. I was entranced. I'll try to give you a picture of what it was like: Every movement that someone made, every gesture, every sound, every light that went on or off, every piece of jewelry, every expression, every type of clothing, every bird that flew by – everything that happened meant something. The beauty and the intensity were unforgettable.

I was admitted to a psychiatric unit and later transferred to a mental institution. The psychiatrist would rush in like the wind each morning with a team of people — a 20-second "hello, how are you?" — and then they were gone. The experts determined that I had chronic undifferentiated schizophrenia. My family was told that I would spend the rest of my life in a hospital; there was no chance of my recovery.

At a time when I most needed to be listened to, understood, validated, and engaged, the seclusion room felt like the worst thing that could have been done to me — isolated in a locked, barren room with bars on the windows. My mind was in a deep fog from the psychiatric drugs. I would hide the pills in my cheek and then spit them out. They changed me to liquid medication. I did what I had to do to get out of the hospital and go back to life on the outside. I was not sure what life would look like, but at least I'd be out of the asylum.

Over 30 years later, I continue to find answers and meaning in what happened to me at the age of 16. I have worked in a psychiatric village in rural Senegal, and at the major psychiatric hospital for West Africa. I've gotten to see mental health programs all across the U.S. I've run group homes, case management programs, recovery education groups, and housing programs for people labeled with mental illness.

It has taken me many years to realize that what was labeled as "chronic schizophrenia" was really a spiritual breakthrough. My mind was not going through the usual cognitive process, but instead reaching out for a deep sense of meaning and purpose in a world that wasn't making sense. I don't know if I was reaching for spirit or it was reaching for me. All I know is that it was overpowering, it was something I couldn't ignore, and it was front and center in my life for a good reason. The awakening I went through then still resonates within me today. This experience very much determined the pathway of my life.

On May 12th, 1971, at about six o'clock,
everything suddenly and unexpectedly
changed.

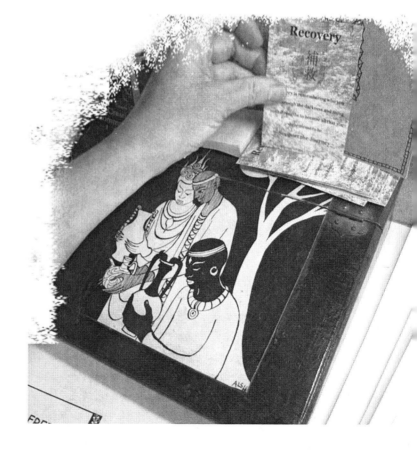

Lauren, is there a particular place where you'd like to start?

I'll start from the beginning. I was born in Washington, D.C., in 1956. My mother used to tell me that I came out so quickly, she almost didn't make it into the delivery room. I grew up in a very stable middle class neighborhood. Appearance was very important; my mother loved for everything to look beautiful and in order. I was, without question, the best-dressed kid in my elementary school. There was almost no hugging or warm emotional expression. I never saw my parents touch one another. Ever.

Life just went on and one day on May 12th, 1971, at about six o'clock, everything suddenly and unexpectedly changed. I was putting a Jefferson Airplane album on down in the basement and I heard a knock at the door. My mother screamed – something I had never heard before. I rushed upstairs and she was surrounded by two men in dark suits. She said, "Your father has been shot."

This started the long wait. The world stopped and nothing of any significance was happening, except that my father was still breathing after the bullet was removed from his brain. I didn't go to school. We spent our days at the hospital. On May 28th, never having regained consciousness, my father died, and the world as I knew it ended. I struggled to wrap my mind around it. This was my first experience in not being able to believe reality. I was 14 and a half – what kind of world was this?

You couldn't admit that he really died?

He was murdered by a teenager with a handgun. Back then, that kind of violence didn't happen to people who lived in the middle class suburbs. It was crushingly sad, but I started school again in the fall, and after about a year and a half, I began feeling like my life went on. On the outside I was looking pretty good, I did what I thought a typical adolescent would do: have fun, make friends, do well in school, do the dishes, keep putting one foot in front of the other. The routine of life had returned.

I had a perfect 16th birthday, spending the night on Old Rag Mountain. I fell in love with a boy I met on the mountaintop. Being in love was new to me – I had never felt such intensity of positive emotions. I started needing less sleep and feeling like something was going on that I didn't quite understand. One day, late in the afternoon, 16 days after my 16th birthday, I started having very strong feelings about wanting to clean up the streets from the murderers and the drug dealers.

Change the world...

Yes, change the world. I didn't believe in God at the time. I didn't believe in a God that would cause the Vietnam War or my father's murder. But I felt like God had picked me to do something special – to rid the streets of drugs and crime. That evening, these feelings became very intense, very strong.

I was a tea kettle that was simmering and simmering... and then suddenly the heat was turned up. I walked through my neighborhood just after sunset. I was alone. I felt the presence of a higher power rapidly growing in intensity, embracing me, and invading every cell of my body. It was extraordinary. I wanted to follow where it was leading me because it felt so right. I decided to tell my mother that I needed her help to reach the President of the United States.

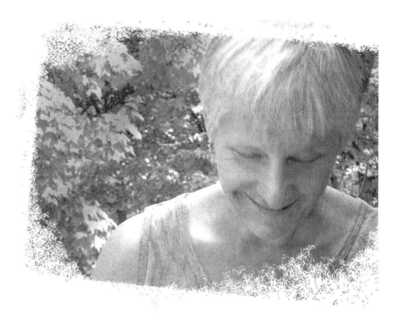

My mother took me to a psychiatrist the next day. He determined I needed to go straight to the hospital psychiatric unit. I was admitted right there in Silver Spring and that was my start on this journey.

Did it feel right that you were there?

No, no. A lot of it wasn't right! I've had over 30 years to think about what happened, and why, and how could it have been different. When I look back now, I think if I had received appropriate services, I did not need to be in a mental institution. What I needed was for someone to trust that my mind was intact. I needed someone who had faith in me to engage me in dialogue, to be with me, and to validate me. I needed someone to help me focus, slow down my thoughts, and be present. My "delusions" were recordings of where my thoughts and emotions were stuck. I needed someone to say: "Why is this happening now? What's going on now? How does it feel? What do you want to do?" I did not need to be hospitalized. The insurance company did not need to spend $200,000.

At the hospital, the drugs weighed me down and made me sluggish. My vision was so blurry, I couldn't read. It was hard to walk. We had private insurance so I assumed I was getting the best treatment money could buy. I trusted the professionals and my parents. Why wouldn't I? I was put on very high doses of anti-psychotic medication. Nothing worked. So they put me on higher and higher doses.

The bottom for me was the night I spent in a seclusion room alone, locked up, drugged up. I remember the feeling that my spirit and soul were being killed. What was left of me, this tiny flickering light, was being extinguished. The walls were solid; the window was sealed with bars. All I had was one hospital gown and a mat on the floor. That was the night I gave myself permission to end my life.

In a nine-by-nine-foot square, white, barren cell, I stood in hell: flames burning, voices screaming, thoughts racing, people laughing, God speaking. It was the lowest place one could go: isolated, alone in a cage within a cage, sealed with a stamp of "sickness." After that night, it made sense to me to really put all my effort and energy, every ounce, into trying to find a life worth living. Eventually I stopped listening to the voices. I just said, "I can't do this anymore," and eventually they stopped.

Eventually I stopped listening to the voices; I just said, "I can't do this anymore." And eventually they stopped.

That's interesting. The voices stopped because you stopped them.

My friend and mentor, Dan Fisher, says that when people get more in touch with their own voice, then those other voices stop. The voices just diminish in their intensity and frequency. Learning to believe in ourselves, hear our own voices, and be in our own bodies, the other voices will go away.

When you got out of the hospital, what was your life like back home?

My home was like the Brady Bunch on the surface. My mother had gotten remarried, and my new step-siblings were the same ages as us. Imagine six teenagers living together. If each of us had only one friend over… we're talking 12 teens in the house at the same time. We had three phone lines, which we used to answer saying, "Grand Central!" A lot of parties were going on. But no one in my family, even to this day, has ever asked me, "What was it like in the mental hospital? What happened to you? Why did it happen?"

The message at home was: *Don't say anything. Don't ask Lauren anything.* I didn't have a safe place to talk about what had happened and people were too afraid to ask. My family was well-intentioned and they loved me, but they wanted to protect me from stress. No one wanted to be responsible for me going over the edge again.

One day I wheeled my bicycle into my psychologist's office and he said, "Do you want to know what your diagnosis is?" I remember thinking, *I don't want to know what label they put on me.* He had my chart opened and he just pointed to the words. It said "chronic schizophrenia." I was terrified. The movie *Psycho* went through my mind. *What does this mean for my life?* The "experts" told me and my family that I would be on psychiatric medication all my life, and I would live most of my life in a mental institution, and I had no real chance for a life in the community.

It's just so unbelievable.

In my early twenties, I started going to National Institutes of Health as a subject for experiments. The psychiatrist there said that I had bipolar disorder, which (conveniently enough) qualified me to be in a whole bunch of his studies. I did it for the money, but also because I believed it was honorable. I thought, "Let me contribute to advancing research in the field if I can." I was really a guinea pig, a human guinea pig.

What was being a "guinea pig"?

They put drops in my eyes and looked at how I reacted versus a "normal person." They did different experiments. I was on lithium for a few years. One study I was given a shot of pure amphetamine and they would ask me questions, "Do you feel anxious? Happy? Sad?" This went on for hours. I could feel the amphetamine going up into my vein and then it hit my heart… boy it felt good! But then I got sick, nauseous, vomiting. I said, "I really don't feel well. Is there somewhere I can lay down for a little while?" and the psychiatrist said, "No."

Driving home, I was so sick. I remember crying while pulling over and vomiting and thinking, *How low can my life get? I'm sick. The psychiatrist doesn't even care. I can't tell anyone.* I was being a guinea pig and I felt there was no one I could talk to about it; no one that would listen non-judgmentally and understand what I was experiencing.

The next evening I returned to the NIH. Upon arriving, the psychiatrist told me that the substance I was injected with the day before was tainted. I proceeded with the next study, where they put electrodes on my head. It was a double-blind study, so the nurse on the psychiatric unit where I was sleeping assumed that I was a "normal" volunteer. She made disparaging remarks about the "mentally sick" people. I was humiliated. In the middle of the night, I quit the study, I quit being a guinea pig, and I never returned.

What happened with lithium? Have you stayed on psychiatric drugs?

During these many experiments, I asked the psychiatrist, "How will I know when I no longer need the lithium?" He said, "You'll need it the rest of your life." He was wrong.

I was on and off psychiatric drugs for almost 20 years; then one weekend I went to a workshop for people who had been through the mental health system. The workshop was called "re-evaluation counseling" and the leader was a woman named Janet Foner. She believed psychiatric drugs were harmful, and she told me she had gotten off drugs. I thought, *Wait a minute... whoa!!! Drugs really help some people. They helped me.* But here's this woman who's highly respected...

And she was totally anti-drug?

She thought that psychiatric drugs were harmful, and that there were other ways to learn to heal and effectively manage emotions. When I was on lithium for those three years, I was a zombie. I had no feelings at all. That is not human. I try not to put down any particular path people are on, but I do get concerned about the damage that drugs do to our brains and how they limit our ability to think and feel. I have found other ways to manage my emotions. I still work on it, but I don't need psychiatric drugs today and I don't think I will ever. At least I hope.

Probably the single most important gift that I have received on my journey was something Janet said to me a few years later. She was leading a support group and she challenged me by saying, "There was never anything wrong with you."

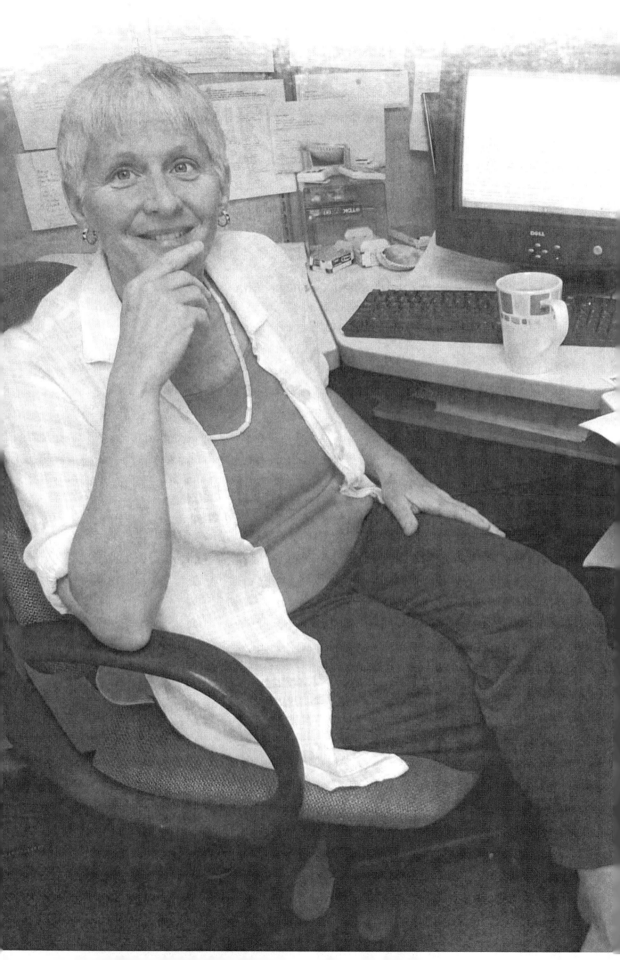

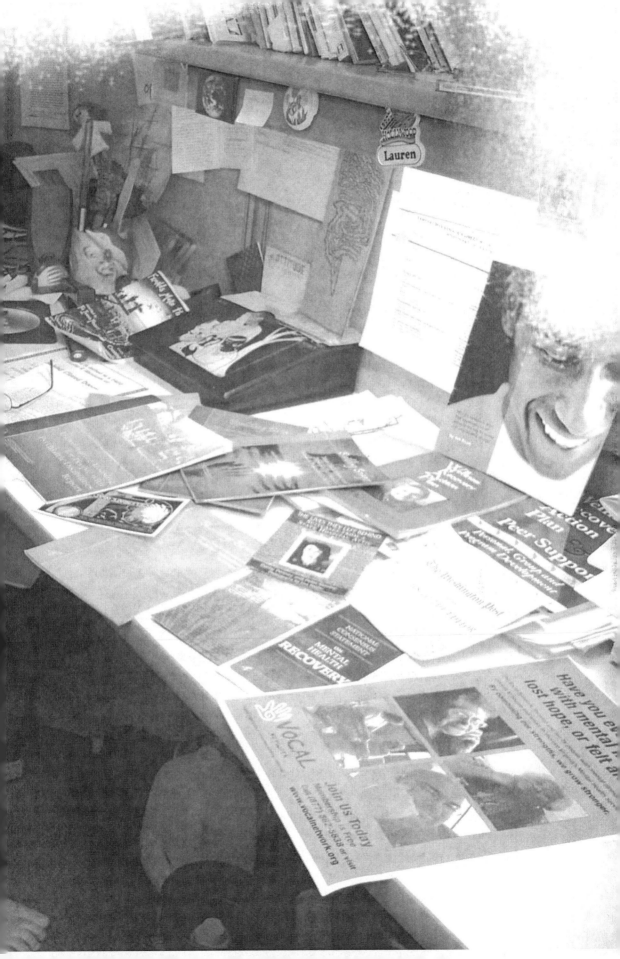

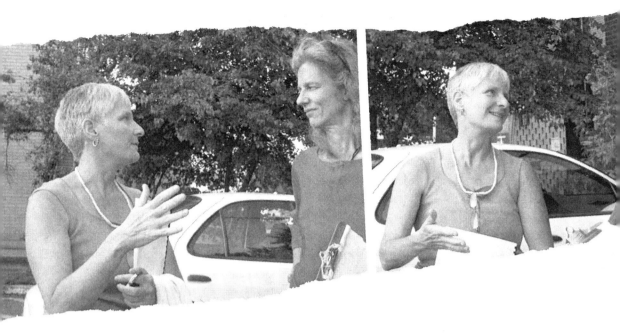

My first response was, "What the hell are you talking about!? What are you thinking? Where are you? There was never anything wrong with me!? I was in a mental institution. I was on psychiatric drugs for years. I've been suffering, mostly in isolation, because I'm afraid to tell anyone that I have this schizophrenia. I'm a freak in this culture and you're telling me there's nothing wrong with me, and there was never anything wrong with me?!"

What if there was never anything wrong with me? She asked me to just stay with that, stay right there. This one question turned my whole thinking inside out. I started to consider the implications. I spent several years trying to reach for something completely different from what I had believed all of my life. *What if society was wrong and what was done to me was wrong? I was a sixteen year old girl whose father had been brutally murdered by a teenager, and I got locked up. What if there was never anything wrong with me? What does it mean? What are the implications for our culture and for our world?*

Did you tell people you had a psychiatric history?

When I went to work in the mental health field, it was the last place in the world I would want people to know that I had been in a mental institution. I was getting promoted at a fairly rapid pace and I was afraid I wouldn't get jobs at the executive level. There's so much discrimination in this field. I did not dare reveal my secret. *Who's going to hire a schizophrenic to run an organization?*

I hid for 30 years.
I was too afraid to tell the truth,
afraid I wouldn't get promoted,
afraid I wouldn't be respected.

Now I don't care.
I'll do what I can to educate you,
to share my journey, to listen to you,
but I'm not going to lie anymore.

For 30 years I kept publicly silent. Then I began my job in Arlington County in the public mental health system. It was a new position: Recovery Advocate and Educator. I started by going across the agency, introducing myself, and speaking about mental health recovery, hope, healing, empowerment, and connection.

But still no disclosure?

I was so naïve. I thought, *I'm a Recovery Advocate and Educator. I was hired to teach people about mental health recovery. I don't need to tell them that I'm a psychiatric survivor myself.*

I started doing the rounds with the different treatment teams – outpatient, dual diagnosis, intensive community treatment. During my first talk, one of the teams said, "Lauren, we've been there; we've done that. We already connect. We already have hope. We're already into recovery and empowerment." A lot of well-intentioned staff people say they get it. They say, "We get it, we get it, we get it." And I listen to them, and from my stance, they don't get it. I realized that I needed to share my story to illustrate for them that they're not doing it the way it needs to be done.

Very quickly, I disclosed… and now my whole life is different. I have this new identity of psychiatric survivor. My friendships have changed; my relationships have changed; my priorities have changed; everything has changed. Some people in my life are moving towards retirement, or retiring, or slowing down. And I'm speeding up.

I hid for 30 years. I was too afraid to tell the truth, afraid I wouldn't get promoted, afraid I wouldn't be respected. Now I don't care. I'll do what I can to educate you, to share my journey, to listen to you, but I'm not going to lie anymore. I'm not going to be silent. That's all part of what it means to know that there was never anything wrong with me.

When I started this job, my first meeting was with eight senior managers, a lot of PhDs. I remember telling them, "I don't intend to duplicate what you are already doing. I'll assume you're doing a good job at helping people function. But underneath the functioning, there is a broken person. My focus is to heal that broken person." One of them said, "Well, that's all of us." I said, "Yes, it is. Exactly."

How did people respond when you started disclosing?

I remember telling my boss that I recovered from being labeled as having chronic schizophrenia and asking him what he thought. He said he thought that I was in "remission" and that the nature of the illness is chronic, though it's great that the symptoms aren't bothering me now. *When you are not having symptoms for 30 years, is that still a remission?*

This is part of the oppression in our culture: If you say you've recovered and that you're well, people don't believe you. There is a part of me that hears that and starts having doubts. *Gee, is there something really wrong with me? Could it happen again?* It's important to listen to people with an open mind, and not label them, and not question their thinking, and not dampen their dreams.

Was there anything you wanted to say about the Peace Corps?

I had to lie to get in. Shortly before I applied someone told me, "If you've spent one night in a loony bin, they won't let you in." So I lied. My principles of integrity superseded my principles of honesty. I took a two-year supply of lithium to Senegal with me (though I never ingested one pill).

The Peace Corps was a way of experimenting in another world. I wanted to know, *Who am I? What am I capable of doing? What am I capable of being?* I was placed in a traditional African village. They might as well have put me in a space capsule and shot me off to another planet.

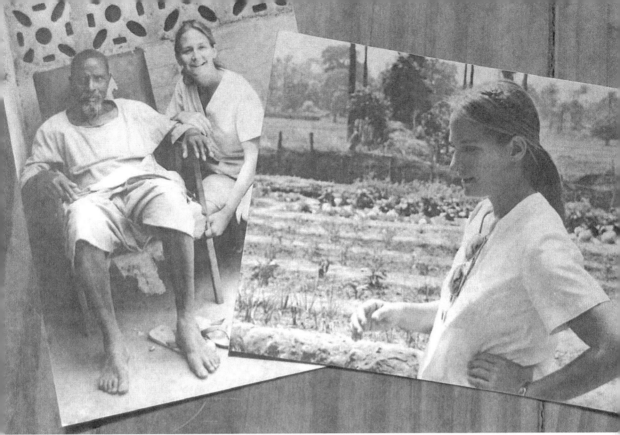

Lauren at 26, in the Peace Corps in Senegal

The early Peace Corps was really the cutting edge of the idealistic volunteer.

Oh God, it was amazing. It was a brilliant idea. What an experience. We had three months of training, and no amount of training could prepare us for what we were facing.

Several people died. Peace Corps volunteers died. A lot of people got very sick, but I wouldn't have given it up for anything. I wanted to live in a world that was very different from white, middle-class, Silver Spring, Maryland. I needed to know that you could think very differently. If you do that in America, they'll lock you up.

What is the Coalition you work with now?

It started when Dan Fisher, the Executive Director of the National Empowerment Center, called a few people around the country to see if they thought it was time to start a national coalition of organizations run by people who have been through the mental health system. I'm sure I gave him the shortest answer of anybody he called. I just said, "Yes. It's time. Let's do it."

We began having national teleconferences, chiseling out a mission statement, and coming up with a name. Dan got a grant to hire someone. One day he called me up and expressed an interest in me applying for the job. I remember the call because he said, "I believe in you." Here is someone I have a great deal of respect for. He is admired by many people around the world, and he says he believes in me.

I wasn't looking for a job. I had never considered this kind of work: going to Capitol Hill and being the face of psychiatric survivors in Washington. People on the teleconferences said, "This is not just a person we hire; this is our voice and our face." It was true, but I thought, "I'm not that person." I didn't believe that I could do such a big job. I started researching the position. I went on the Hill. I talked to people. I used re-evaluation counseling sessions, where I would shake and I would cry – really cry deeply – and let the feelings of terror come up. I thought, *I'm not an extroverted person; I'm not a particularly articulate person; I struggle to find words; I'm an artist who would rather paint it than say it.*

Even after two months, I still didn't know. Two days before the interview I realized that the only thing keeping me back was that I didn't believe in myself. So I made a commitment, a promise to myself. My commitment was: *From this moment on I joyfully promise to believe completely in myself and my ability to listen, learn, love, laugh and be a light of transformation.*

Now, thirty-one states belong to the National Coalition of Mental Health Consumer/Survivor Organizations and I'm the Director of Public Policy. The first and (for now) only staff person.

What was your daily life like when you were at your lowest point and what is your daily life like now?

Well, at 16 I was locked in a mental institution. I was very confused and mostly numb from the drugs. I put one foot in front of the other and did what I was told to do.

And now?

My daily life now is more exciting, meaningful, and gratifying than it has ever been. No two days are alike on the Coalition job. I am meeting senators, congressmen and congresswomen, staffers, and leaders from other national organizations. I'm serving on planning committees, putting out press releases, and speaking at conferences. I speak with providers, policy makers, and law and medical school students. Our Steering Committee includes the directors of three national mental health assistance centers, so that we can work in a coordinated way to build our voice.

Our Coalition co-sponsored two presidential candidate forums, one in New Hampshire and one in Ohio. Ted Kennedy Jr. moderated the first forum. He and Hillary Clinton electrified the room. I was telling Ted (whose wife is a psychiatrist) about how I had recovered from being labeled with chronic schizophrenia. His reaction was one I frequently hear, "I've never heard that people can recover from mental illness." When I hear someone say that, I get to explain, "That is why we have a Coalition. We are the voice of people who have recovered, and now we are being heard."

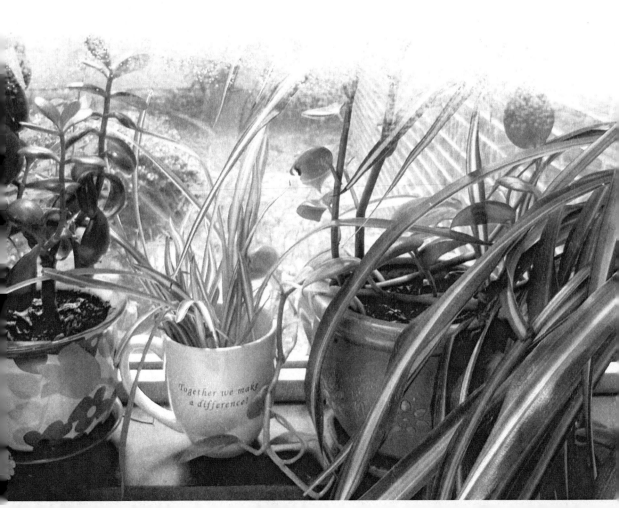

When I was 16, I wanted to reach the President.
Those thoughts were labeled as a delusion,
hallucination, psychotic...

Now it's the work
I'm doing.

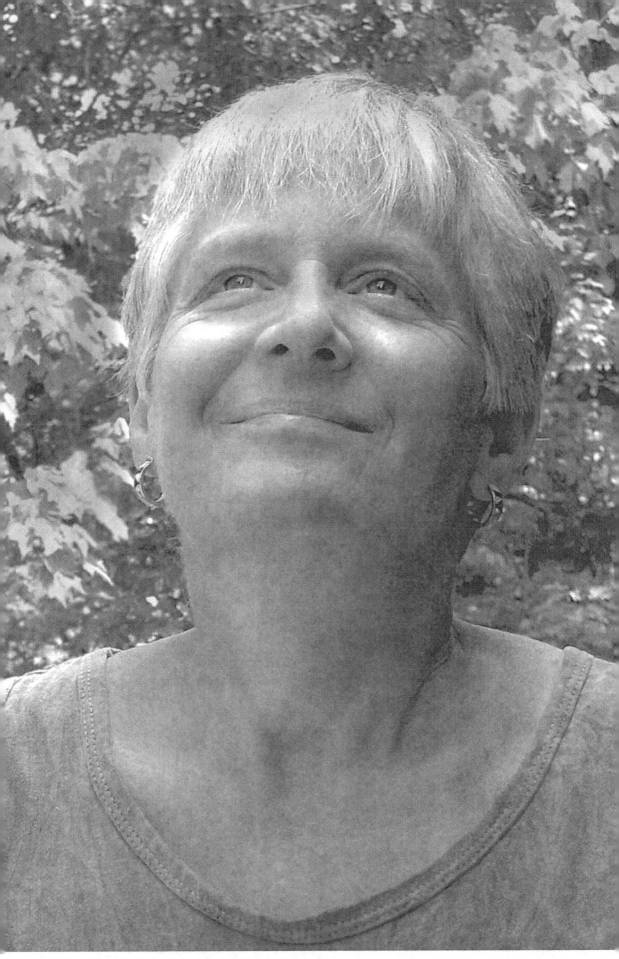

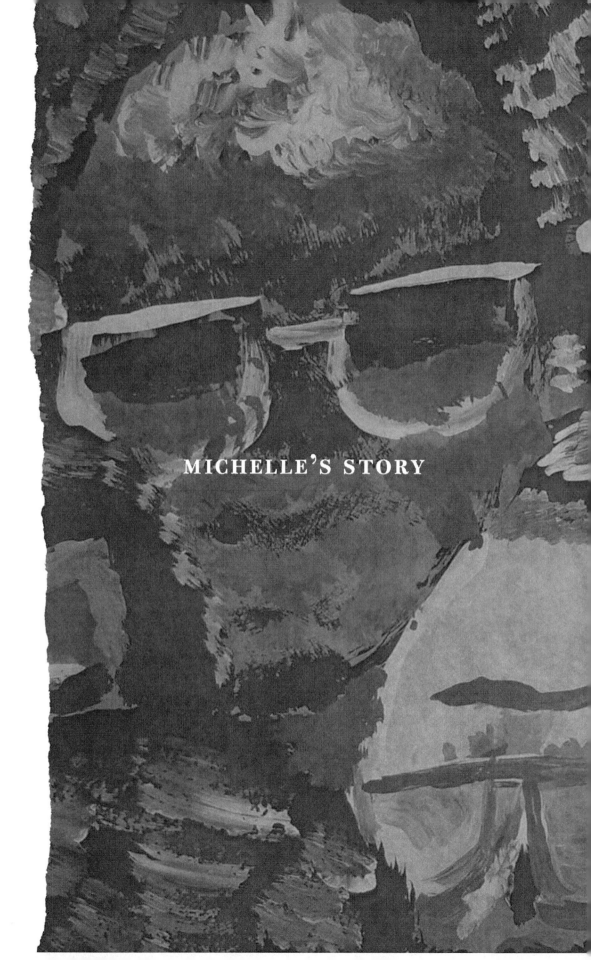

MICHELLE'S STORY

*How has my life been enriched
by mental illness?*

Well, I've met people I never
thought I would meet, I've gone
places I never thought I would
go, I've done things I never
thought I would do.
I've experienced things that
I never in my wildest dreams
thought I would experience.

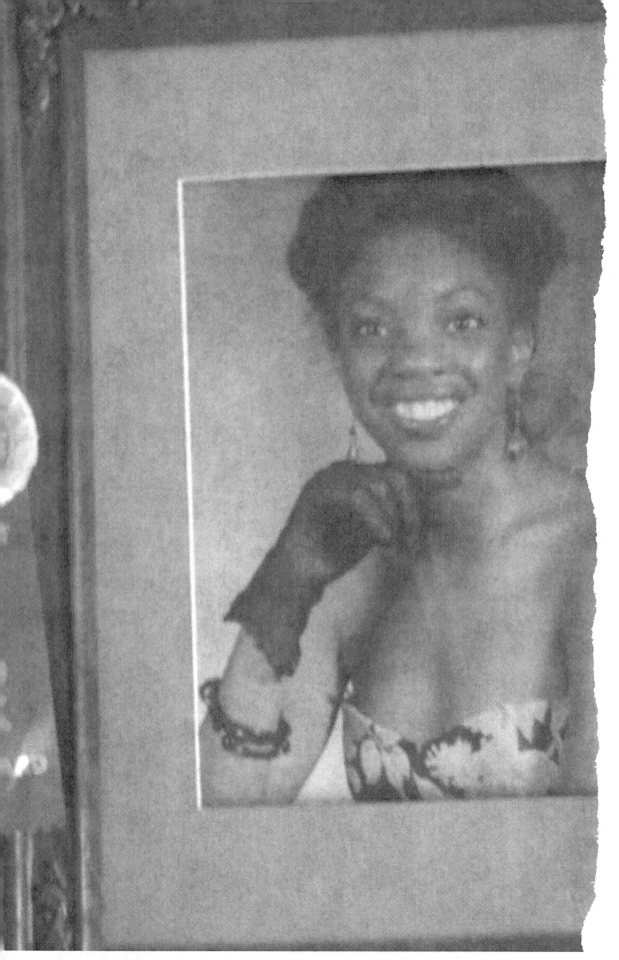

My life

is chapters and chapters of hurt and pain, dark nights and deep flood waters. But mental illness also came with great abilities and incredible gifts. I can draw, paint, write, sing, play piano, dance, do crafts, teach and dream. I can empathize, care, and instill hope. I can see the angels of God and the demons of hell, and I can see the auras that surround people and the color of their mood. Music plays in my head to soothe my soul and Scripture comes to recall when I least expect it. These gifts ease up the darkness in this world and fill me with hope.

I have been homeless and slept in parks and cemeteries. Now I have a home. I have lost my five children to the courts for two years; now I have six. I have been abused by friends and spouses; now I live with my soul mate. I have had nine journeys to the psychiatric ward; now my meds keep me sane. I have been friendless, lost, and out of my mind hallucinating; now I have peers that are real friends, a position as a mental health recovery facilitator, and a loving church family.

At the beginning, I didn't think there was any possibility of recovering from my mental illness and from my brain injury. If there was a hopeless person in the world, it was me. I did everything and anything I could to kill myself and failed at every single attempt.

When I go through a hardship now I think, "I'm going through the fire of this situation, but I can get out on the other end. There will be an end to this. I've just got to wait it out, and I can wait it out." I tell myself, "Once I get out of this depression, I'll be able to take it and use it with the recovery group that I'm teaching or with a particular person that I'm trying to help at the vocational center."

I can go up to someone now and say, "OK, I've worn those shoes, I've worn that hat, I know where you're coming from. Let's take it from here. Let me stand beside you. Let me hold your hand and help you walk through this so that you're not walking alone."

Interviews by Debra Knighton, Bev Ball, Mitzi Ware & Cynthia Power;
Photographs by Cassandra Nudel

Michelle, how does your story begin?

I had signs that there was something odd about myself since I was a kid. Not to scare you, but I could see demons and I could see angels all around me. I couldn't tell whether I was looking at a person or an angel or a demon. Different people would have different colors around them based upon what their mood might be – mostly it was bright colors like red or orange or yellow or pink or white. My mom would say, "Don't talk about that. Don't tell people that."

When I was a teenager, one of my brothers got into trouble with the law. Once the newspaper published the address, everybody knew it was our family. We had difficulty at school after that. The kids were really cruel to my brothers and me. As a result of that situation, I was raped by two guys from my work, a classmate and the swing-shift manager. I kept it to myself, but shortly after that, I started having psychiatric symptoms.

I wouldn't go to school. I wouldn't go outside. I wouldn't go to work. I was 16 and I was basically catatonic on my bed. When my father had had enough, he came into my room and yelled in my face, trying to get me to snap out of it. He dressed me and put me on the school bus. I went back to school, but I couldn't stop crying. I would go to school crying, spend the whole day crying, and come home crying. The school decided to let me finish out my last two years in the counselor's office. My teachers brought my schoolwork to me. My parents thought I was just being an emotional teenager. Here they had a daughter that spent most of her time crying, and they just ignored me.

Once I got to college, I really went "off the hook." I wouldn't go to classes, except to take the tests. I would go to the campus sanctuary and sing and study my Bible, or I would go to the library and read books, and write notes that made no sense at all. I spent no time with people. One day I went to the circle in the center of the College grounds, stood on top of the wall and began to preach fire and brimstone to everybody passing by. I thought I was the prophet Jeremiah and they were all going to go to hell except for me. The school let that go on for about a month.

One snowy evening, they found me outside in my nightgown crying. They put me on a bus and sent me back home.

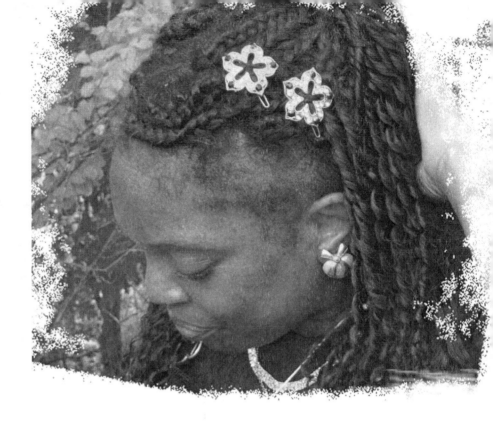

One snowy evening,
they found me outside
in my nightgown crying.

Can you tell us a story about fire?

A story of a fire I went through: It started when I was in a car accident on April 11th, 1997. I was in a semi-coma for three days. When the doctors tested me, they said I was on a third grade level. That was when I finally got diagnosed. They came to the conclusion that I had both a mental illness and a brain injury. I had to learn how to walk, to climb, to bend, to sit. I had to learn to feed myself again; I had to learn to write again; I had to learn to use a dishwasher and a washer and dryer. I mean, I had to learn *everything* all over again.

Having a brain injury is really interesting. The first time I saw rain I thought the sky was falling. I flipped out. I really thought the sky was falling. I had to learn that water falling from the sky is rain and it's normal. Seeing a tree sway back and forth blew me away, because I thought the trees were falling, but I found out they're not falling. They're swaying back and forth.

I was married at the time. My husband hung in there for about a year, then one day he called a taxi and just left us. After he left, social services told me that I could apply for disability benefits, but if I did they would take my kids. They said the only other route was to get a job, take care of my kids, and go on a government assistance program called TANF (Temporary Aid for Needy Families). That's what I did.

I found out TANF does not work. I'll let that be known, TANF does not work! I did TANF for a short time, then I got off it and worked three jobs to take care of my five kids. At the same time, I went through physical therapy, speech therapy and cognitive therapy. I asked my father if he would help me take care of my children and he said, "You made your bed and you sleep in it." He wanted nothing to do with anybody who had a mental health disability, and he wanted nothing to do with me. I was on my own for a very long time. I literally didn't sleep for years.

At that point I made a really bad decision. Working three jobs and not getting any sleep started to catch up with me. I knew I was getting sick; I felt it inside. When you have hallucinations, you see things that aren't there. You know they aren't there and you try to keep from reacting, but you can't help it – so you react and it scares everybody around you. It was getting really hard just to go to work and be among people. So, I chose to just out-and-out marry this person who I'd only known for three months. He went to the church I belonged to at that time. I thought, *Well, he goes to the church I go to, and everybody knows him, so if anything happens, people will be there to rescue me.* It was a very bad decision. The first thing he did was put me in the mental hospital.

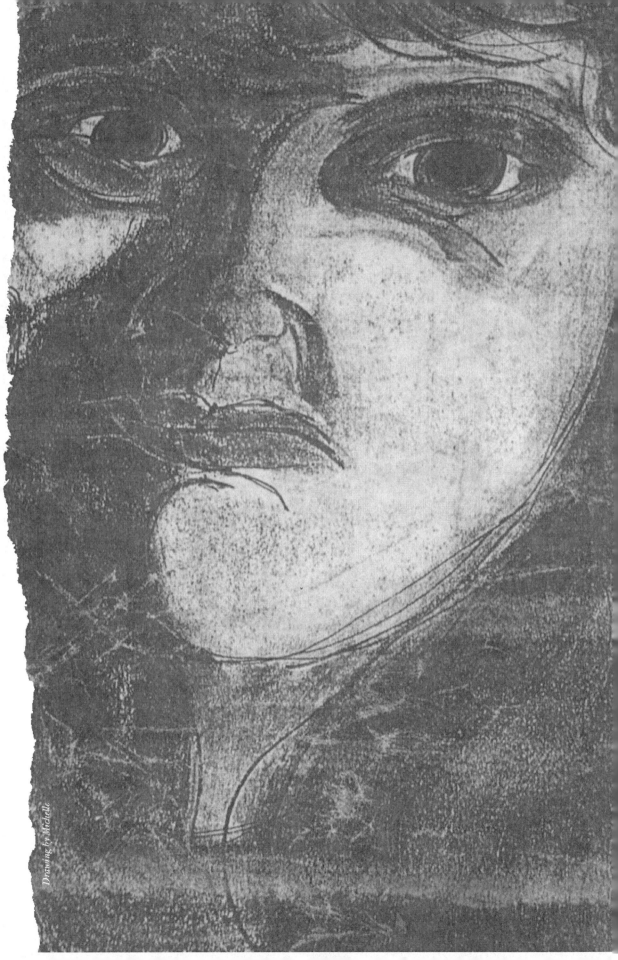

When I came out, they put me on high doses of medication. I was a zombie all day long. My husband basically got me out of bed, dressed me, fed me, sat me by the window and turned on the TV. That's where I lived for six months.

I learned a hard lesson: If you get a diagnosis, you have to educate yourself about what they're telling you. Find out if the medication works for you and how high the dosage needs to be. When they sent me home on a high dose of medication, to them I was stable and that made them happy. Half my life is gone. I don't know anything about that time, because I was so "stable."

I spent six months staring into space. The wake up call came in June of 2002, when the police broke into our house and arrested my then-husband and marched my five children out of the house and did not tell me where they went. There was an investigator breathing down my throat saying, "You know everything that was going on!" I said, "I don't know anything. I don't know." Eventually they found that I truly didn't know anything, and they let me go. It turned out my ex-husband was a criminal. He is still in prison today for the crimes he committed.

That was one of my darkest periods of going through the fire. It scared the daylights out of me. I got off the medication and refused to take it again. I closed myself into the house by myself and just went off the deep end. I remember going from one hallucination to the other, thinking that my kids were there when I knew they weren't.

I have been homeless and slept in parks and cemeteries. Now I have a home. I have lost my five children to the courts for two years; now I have six.

Where were your kids at that point?

I would see my kids like phantoms. Part of me believed they were there with me; part of me believed they were dead.

They were with my dad, but I didn't know at the time, so I was constantly searching for them. I would call up my dad begging, "Please, where are my kids? Tell me where my kids are!" and he would hang up the phone. I would go to different people's homes from my past church, and I would bang on their doors, yelling, "Please give me my kids!"

I built a cemetery in the backyard. I made a plot for each one of my kids and each one of my husbands. I would go out there every day and visit the cemetery and talk to my kids. My neighbor kept reporting to the police that someone needed to take care of this lady, because I was scaring her. A couple of times her husband went out there and took the cemetery apart, and I just went out and put it back together. There were times that I slept out there. To me, I was with my family out there.

Eventually my landlord hired a man to take care of the property – because I wasn't taking care of it at all. Keith would come over and take care of the house and the yard, and then he would come into the house. I would be taking glasses out of the cabinet and throwing them on the floor and shattering them and screaming. He'd just stand behind the door and wait for me to finish and then he'd come in with a broom and clean up. Then he'd go into the living room and sit where I was and just wait for me to start talking to him for the day. That was Keith.

It sounds like that was a turning point.

That was the biggest turning point. Keith had no reason under the sun to have anything to do with me whatsoever. I got so bad I wasn't eating, I wasn't bathing, I wasn't dressing and I just wasn't taking care of myself. I was totally sick, completely out of my mind, off the deep end. Yet he hung in there with me. He would just spend the day with me and make sure that I didn't hurt myself.

Keith was afraid that eventually I was going to kill myself, so he tried different things to get me out of the house. This one particular Valentine's Day, after I had drunk five bottles of white wine, we were crossing the Rappahannock Bridge, and I had the delusion that if I could just fly off the bridge, I could get to my kids. I jumped out of the car, ran across three lanes of traffic, and almost jumped off the bridge. Keith ran across three lanes of traffic after me. To anybody who was on the bridge that day: I'm sorry that I the caused traffic, but I almost made it off that bridge and he caught me just in time and pulled me back.

There was a police officer there, and they took me to the hospital. Once I dried out and began taking medication, my head cleared up and I realized, "There's something really, *really* wrong, and if I don't do something now I'm going to die." I finally made the decision that I was going to start taking responsibility for myself and for my life.

One of the first things I did was ask, "Do I have to take the medication that

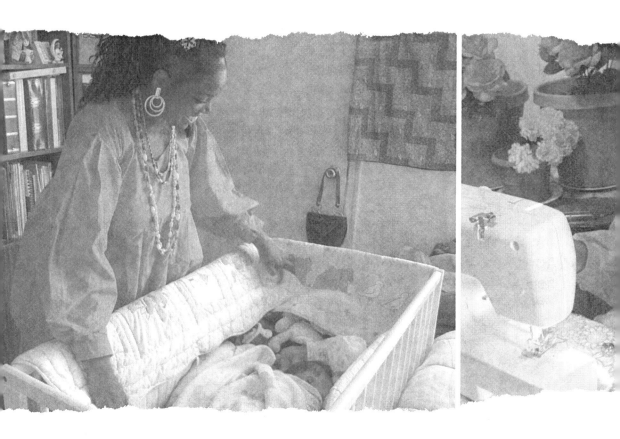

you suggest, or can I suggest medication for myself?" They said, "If you think there's something else that might work for you, be our guest." They gave me a medication booklet and a pill book to look through. We chose some medications and tried them and they worked well for me.

I had a therapist named Brandy who believed in recovery from mental illness. Instead of asking, "Are you taking your medication?" she would ask, "What do you want to do with your life?" That was the beginning of my recovery.

I want to hear about you getting your children back. You just kept going to court and eventually got them back?

I would go to court, and I would say, "What do I need to do to get my kids?" And they would say, "We want you to go to parenting classes." I would take every single parenting class I could find, then I would go back to court and say, "OK, I took parenting classes. Now what?" They would say, "We want you to be on your medication for a good nine months before we consider you." So I was on my medication for nine months consistently. "Now we want you to try

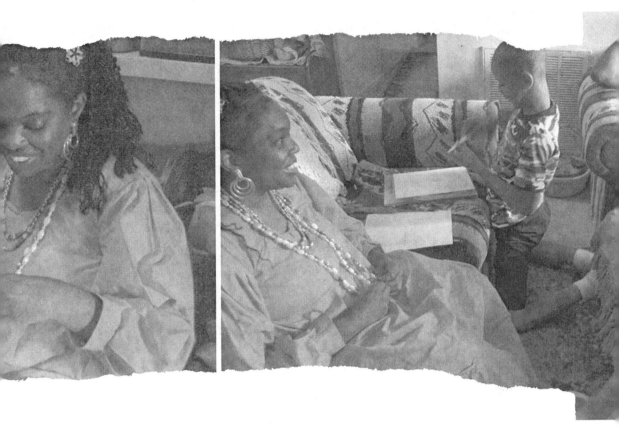

to build a relationship with the children's grandfather (my dad) and visit the kids every so often." So I did all that, and they said, "Now we want to see you outside of the house more." The vocational center helped me do that. Finally the court said, "You have proven that you have a stable home life, so we're going to give the kids back to you."

If you have been diagnosed with a mental illness and you lose your children, it's a hard road to get your kids back, but I did get them back. My children have been with me since January of 2004. My children don't need to go to foster care. They don't need to go to different family members. They can stay with me, and I can take care of them.

What happened with Keith?

I made Keith wait five years before I married him. I did the right thing marrying Keith. I married my soul mate. He's just incredible and he doesn't see that in himself. He is the most trustworthy person on the planet and extremely kind. I could not be without Keith. He brought a lot of stability. He brought the quietness and the peace.

How did your daily life at your lowest point compare with your daily life now?

I never poured into a cup — I just drank from bottle after bottle. I just sat in a stupor thinking of the many ways I could commit suicide and how sorry everybody would feel once they found me.

The last few years have been mostly quiet and calming. I've been concentrating on my girls and my boys. I've been concentrating on my new husband Keith, helping him get strong the way he helped me get strong. Now I am a mental health recovery facilitator; I'm becoming a peer support specialist; I'm advocating on behalf of my peers at the vocational center.

How did your family react when you were diagnosed?

I have a sister-in-law who will literally get in my face and say, "HOW ARE YOU TODAY?!" She limits everything to a second-grade level. "HOW... DID... YOUR... DAY... GO... MICHELLE?... DID... YOU... EAT... TODAY?... VERY.... GOOD!" My family believes that people who have been diagnosed with mental illness are retarded. It's just their opinion and I accept that. There is no changing their mind.

My biological family abandoned me. It really hurts to say that, but I have to be honest. My dad's reaction was that I needed to stop taking the medication, get myself together, start driving again, get myself a government job and just accept the way life is, because life is tough. Right now, I lead mental health recovery groups, and I am getting trained to become a mental health peer support specialist. I told my family that I'm going to work for the county, but they think I'm under a delusion, that this is a "made-up fantasy of Michelle's."

I love them to death. They are my family. They gave birth to me and I grew up with them, but I have found that it is better to avoid them. I don't think it's uncommon. I can't say they're doing something no other family has done. I hope other families will read this book and use it as a tool. I'm hoping that I can give it to my family and they'll take the time to read it and begin treating me like a person.

My biological family has no hope for me whatsoever... on the other end of the totem pole, my friends and my church family have all the hope in the world. They care about me and they love me and they were there for me the whole time. That's family.

When I first came to church, I had some odd ways. They didn't mind. I would sit out in the foyer by myself because I was so agoraphobic, so afraid of people touching me, people being near me, people getting to know me. The church put up speakers in the foyer so that I could hear the service. This one family would take turns sitting out there with me. Eventually I started singing with the choir, but as soon as the singing was over, I'd go back to the foyer and people would come and sit with me. They did that with me for two years until I felt comfortable enough to sit in the sanctuary with everybody else.

When I was in the psychiatric hospital, my church family still called and visited. They said, "When people get sick, they go into the hospital. You're going to get out and things will be fine." A few times I've had panic attacks at church, and it hasn't been a problem. My church friends dealt with it, and they calmed me down. They took me in and accepted me and loved me, and that has kept me out of the hospital.

My church family is there for me 100%. They're there to help me in whatever I need; they don't ask questions, and they trust me. I give them my life and my heart, and I tell them, "Thank you. You are the reason why I'm still standing here." I didn't write myself off, because they didn't write me off.

Instead of asking,
"Are you taking your medication?"
she would ask,
"What do you want to do with your life?"
That was the beginning of my recovery.

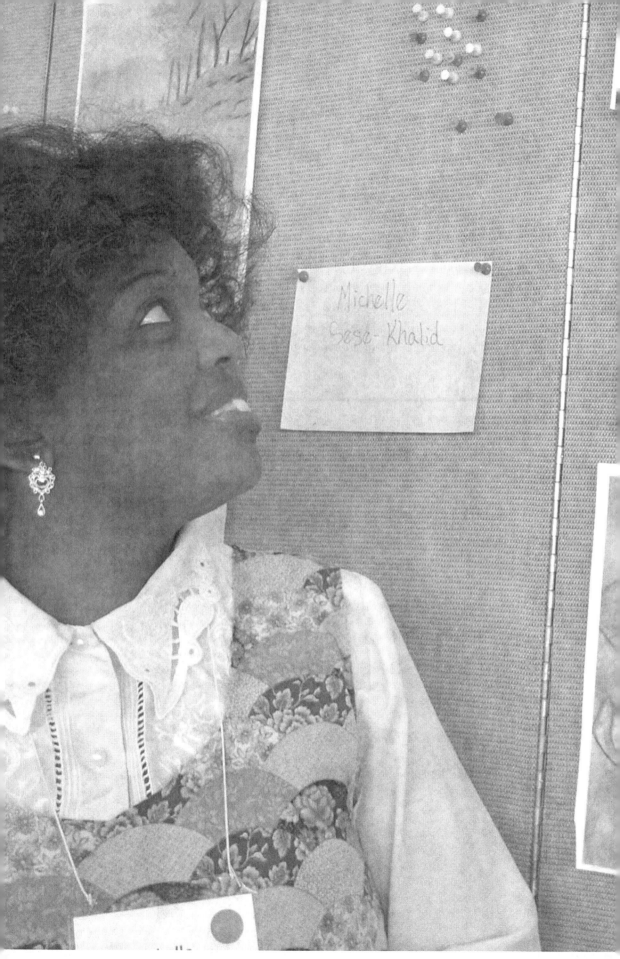

Michelle
Sese-Khalid

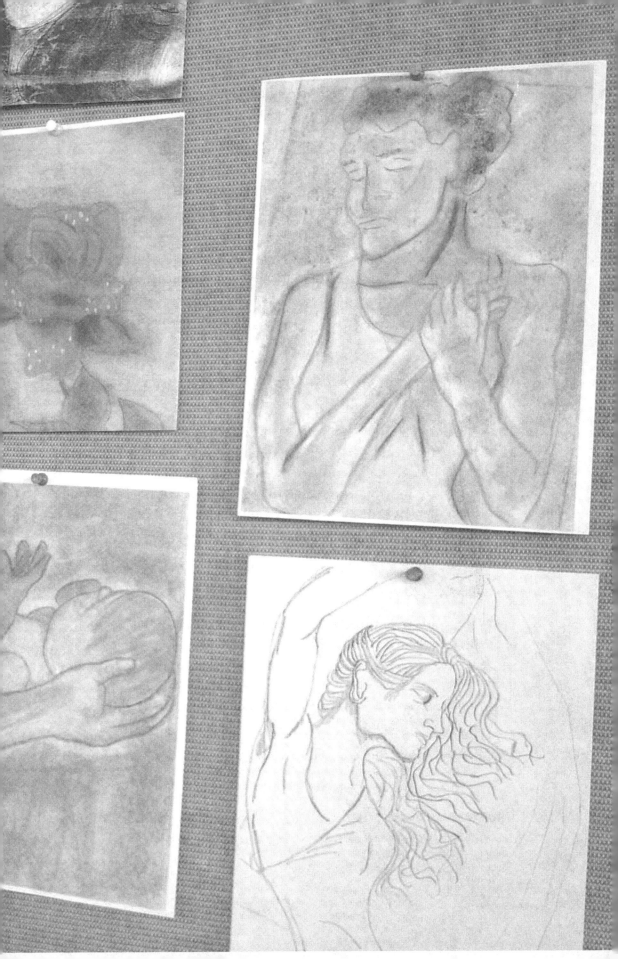

How do mental health and recovery fit into your world view and your belief system?

I'm not embarrassed to say that I'm a born-again Christian. No, I don't speak in tongues. No, I don't get into being "slain in the spirit." I'm a conservative Baptist. I do believe in studying my Bible, and I do believe in the power of prayer. That keeps me on my feet in this life, and I know that I have a place that I will go when I die.

I think the *Firewalkers* book is very important in Christian circles. A lot of times people in the Christian church believe mental health symptoms are the result of sin in your life. I'm here to say: No, I'm not demon-possessed. No, there is not sin in my life. I have a disease of the brain, but I can overcome it.

Is there part of your faith that has been something for you to hold onto in the dark times?

The way I pray is I sing. The words are like God's love letter saying, "You're in the palm of my hand; I'm not going to let you fall." When the depression hits and I feel like I can't get out, and the darkness is going to swallow me up, sometimes it's really hard to have courage to get up and walk outside the room and meet the day. Music has a way of strengthening me and making me want to stand up and be firm and consistent and courageous.

You've talked a little about being angry with God.

I'm 39. I'm getting a little older, a little more mature, a little wiser. Those angry outbursts towards God went from being, "I don't want to talk to you because you let this happen," to "Why did you let this happen?" then to "OK, these things happened. Where am I going to go from here? You allowed me to go through these situations. Now what's the point? Show me the point."

I didn't understand where everything was going, but here I am four years later, and I look back and I think, *Ah, now I see!*

If you could go back in time and magically change your life so that you never experienced mental health struggles, would you do it?

Ten years ago, I would have said, "Yes!" and pleaded with you to do something about me. My mind, my thoughts, and my emotions scared me and others. It was exhausting, tiring, maddening.

But would I still want to change myself now? No. I like being eccentric. I like who I am right now. I like the fact that I can relate to the hurt and the pain and the sadness that other people go through. Mental health struggles are a gift God has given me so that I can care about other people and not be so self-absorbed. I don't want to be like everybody else. That's the way He made me, and that's the way it is. No changing.

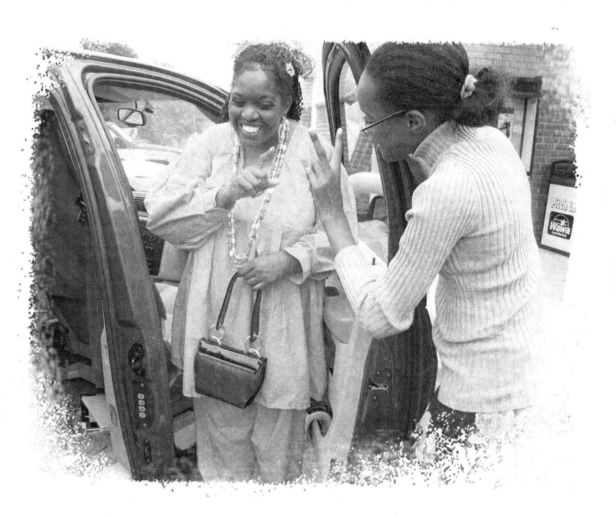

I can go up to someone now and say,

"OK, I've worn those shoes, I've worn that hat, I know where you're coming from. Let's take it from here. Let me stand beside you. Let me hold your hand and help you walk through this so that you're not walking alone."

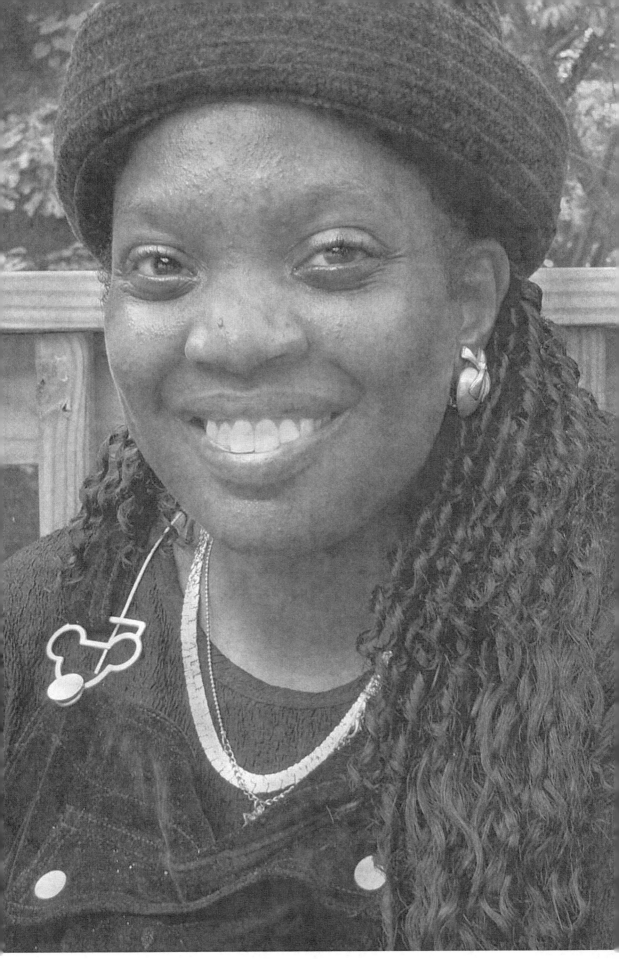

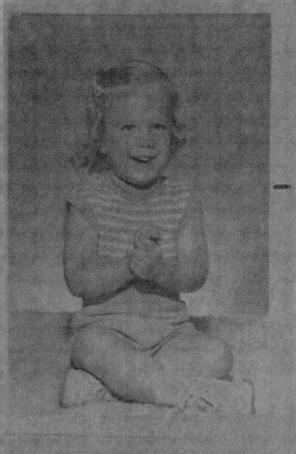

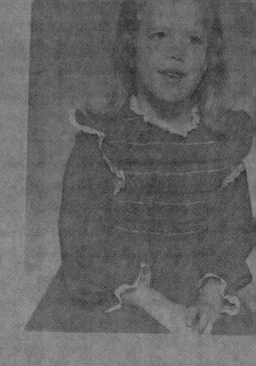

DEBRA'S STORY

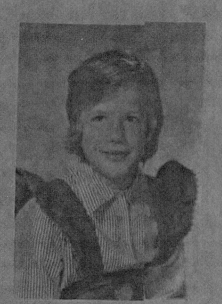

4th grade

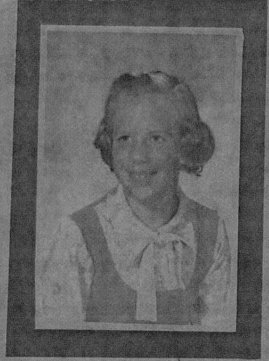

3rd grade

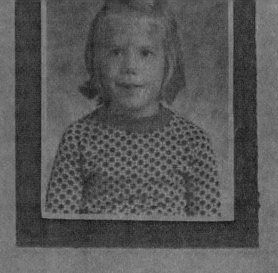

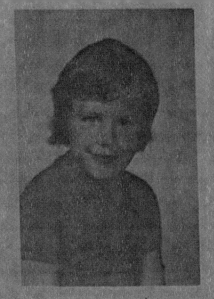

2nd grade

My story starts at age twelve.
I was a smart, chubby pre-teen.

5th grade

The boys at the swimming pool called me
"Minnie" (short for "Minnesota Fats").

6th grade
1981

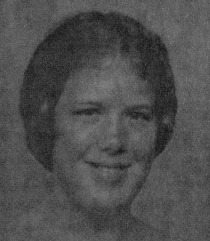

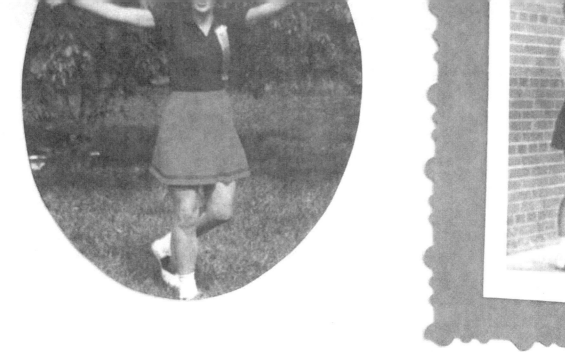

Debra was a cheerleader her Junior &
Senior year. She was an alternate her
Junior year & the school mascott (the Bee) her senior year.
She won the incentive award her junior year (for
displaying a good attitude & putting forth a lot of effort).

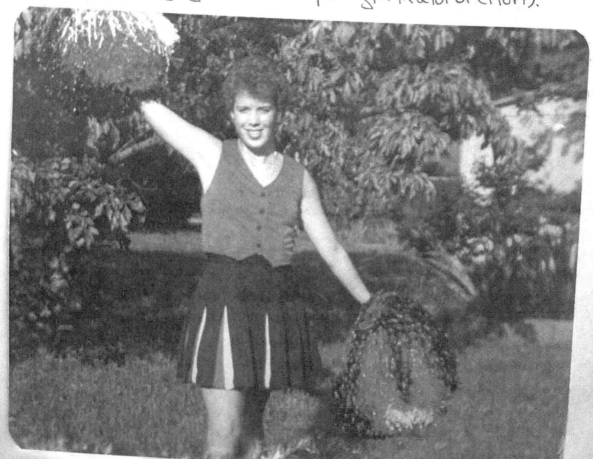

When

I turned 15 and decided to lose weight, I quickly dropped 40 pounds through diet and exercise. I would exercise whenever my parents left the house. I binged on cereal and exercised like mad to burn off the calories. By the time I got to college, I was deep into bulimia. I dealt with stress by binging, purging, cutting, banging my head against the wall, and sleeping the day away. I waited tables at two different restaurants and spent my time between jobs binging and purging in the car. I was hospitalized for the first time in the middle of my second year of college, and I've been a part of the mental health system ever since.

I was definitely one of those people who could have stayed in the hospital forever. Whenever I couldn't cope with life outside the hospital, I ended up overdosing or doing something else to land myself back in the hospital where I felt safe from the world and from myself. I eventually became hospital-dependent.

My mom always used to say, "People won't like you if you're not happy. People won't want to be around you if you're not smiling." So I always thought that was why I didn't have any friends. I wasn't happy and people don't like people who aren't happy. In my years growing up, I didn't have intimate relationships.

Then when I was in the hospital, people liked me even though I wasn't happy all the time. I found levels of connection that I hadn't known existed. After I came out, I had more friends than I ever could have imagined – friends from the hospital, friends from my eating disorder group, friends from Overeaters Anonymous, friends from school. Relationships that had been superficial gained depth as we began to relate at a real level around our need for each other and our desire for meaning and purpose.

When I read about Blue Ridge House, I thought, "Wow. That would be a great place for me to do a student internship. They help people with mental health diagnoses get back out into the community. They believe what I believe. Surely if no one else wants me, they would be fine to hire me." Then I got there, and shared my own mental health struggles, and the Director said, "I don't think so." He didn't want me there, but eventually I won him over as I began to connect to members in meaningful ways. In the next few years, I would go from student intern, to volunteer, to part-time worker, to full-time employee.

My mental health struggles have taught me that it's impossible to really know what's going on in someone else's life, so it's important to give them grace. For the most part, people want to be cared about and accepted, regardless of what their actions indicate. When I'm experiencing symptoms, I'm generally not in a place where I can nicely ask for help. I tend to be paranoid and irritable, but I still want to be loved and accepted even when I'm acting like I don't care. When I'm going through my hardest times, what I need most is for people to like me anyway. When other people are having a hard time, that's who I want to be: I want to be that person who likes them anyway.

If I hadn't experienced mental illness, I think I would have had a very small frame of reference. I think I would have been a teacher; I think I would have gone to church; I would still be interacting mostly on a superficial level. I've learned along the way that people really desire to relate at a profound level. I've found out that people crave genuine relationships. I think that I push people into being more open; it feels good and creates more connection. That was one of the reasons that I ended up working in the mental health field: It fosters being real and authentic.

Suffering produces perseverance,
which produces character,
which produces hope.

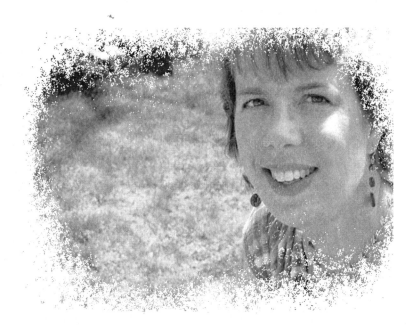

Interviews by Cassandra Nudel, Bev Ball & Ken Moore; Photographs by Cassandra Nudel

Debra, can you tell us about your internal experience with extreme mental states? For some people it's really hard to understand what it feels like from the inside.

When I'm really depressed, I feel angry at the world for requiring me to do anything besides getting out of bed in the morning – or even for requiring me to get out of bed at all. I think about killing myself or wanting to hurt myself. The emotions are just so powerful that it's almost physically painful just to exist. I resent everybody, including my kids and my husband, just because they require *anything* of me. I've been depressed to the point where I don't have the energy to even *think* about killing myself. I feel tired, tired of life, tired of existing. Intellectually I may know that I have a great life and I've been blessed, but it doesn't make any difference during those times.

Then there are times when I'm hypomanic. It's uncomfortable just being *inside myself.* It's really hard when people are looking at me; I know from the outside I look normal. Inside though, everything's raging, my mind is spinning, and it feels like everything is going in a million different directions. I can't rein it in. It feels like my world is just flying apart. There are all these thoughts and voices, and I can't get grounded. It takes a lot of effort and energy to interact with people when everything that is going on in my mind is not related to the conversation I'm having.

It's really sketchy when I have episodes. That's a hard thing for people to understand because it seems like I'm not taking responsibility, but I just don't remember. So I say, "Sure I'm sorry I did that but I don't remember doing that."

I always come out of it. I'm in it for different periods of time, and I come out of it in different ways. The most striking way is a couple of times people have prayed over me and suddenly all the noises in my head cleared – not forever, but for a while, and that was pretty amazing. Sometimes I just have to sleep it off. I am amazed at how what I eat or how often I exercise can affect my thinking and my emotions. When I gave up sugar, I couldn't believe how my energy level surged and emotions lifted. Even more remarkable was the change in my thinking and my mood when I was pregnant and nursing. The hormones were apparently just the right mix for me. It was like a fog lifted that had been there as long as I could remember.

Your experience in the hospital sounds more positive than many other stories. Do you think the difference is that you were in a private hospital not a state hospital?

I think it was more that the doctor and staff there were progressive. When I went into the hospital I hated being there, but I loved being there. I felt more secure, appreciated, and cared for there than I ever remembered feeling. All the pressures of the outside world were gone.

I am acutely aware that my life would have taken a very different course had I ended up in a state hospital rather than at a private facility. Given the irrational thought patterns, unstable mood, and self-destructive behaviors I had during college, I probably would have gotten "stuck" in the mental health system.

I've met a lot of people who went into psychiatric hospitals and were told, "You can give up on going to college. You can give up on your goals." My experience was different. The hospital staff just said, "You may have to work harder at this than other people. You might have to study harder than other people. You may need to do more things to take care of yourself. But if it's worth it to you, then we will help you try to get through it."

I've found that people who gave me
grace rather than judgment
ultimately made the biggest difference in my life.

Now I want to be one of those people for others.

I didn't go to football games and I didn't party. I did things to take care of myself and I got through school. I did a lot of cutting and a lot of banging my head against the wall and binging and purging all over campus, but I got through school. At times I thought it was going to kill me. I won't say I have no pleasant memories of college, though it definitely wasn't the best time of my life. But the doctors and staff were willing to stick it out with me.

You graduated from University of Virginia in both psychology and chemistry, and got a Masters up in Boston. Can you share your educational experience?

My chemistry advisor was broken-hearted (to say the least) when I told him chemistry wasn't the direction I was going in my life. I had the highest grades in the chemistry department, but after being in the hospital and having therapy, I was really seeing the value of people and relationships. I just couldn't see myself working in a lab with test tubes for the long term. So I went to Boston University for a distance learning program in psychiatric rehabilitation.

Psychiatric rehabilitation is about helping people set goals for themselves.

I think there is some hope and energy in beginning to move forward (even if you don't reach the end goal). There is hope in feeling, *I'm doing something to overcome. I'm doing something to gain some victory in life, to move towards something that I want. I don't just have to sit here and take medication and chill out in this place where I am right now.* I'm really glad I did this program because it gave me a philosophy for life, too.

I don't remember anything about chemistry now, except that there's a periodic table. That's about all.

Can you tell us about a time when you tried to hold hope for somebody else?

There was a guy who goes to the mental health program where I work. When he first started coming he was depressed and anxious, and wouldn't make eye contact with anybody. He didn't want to be there, didn't want to do anything. He was saying, "I'm living until I die and that's just as good as it's going to get."

I started talking to him about how smart he was, how gifted he was with computers, and what a great guy he was. We talked about his strengths and we talked about medication –I know a lot of people don't think much of medication, but I thought it might help him. He was afraid of taking medication because he thought it might make him feel like a zombie, until he realized that I was on medication and he said, "I want to take what you're taking!"

He thought his only choices were to be a zombie or to be totally depressed all the time. I wanted to give him some hope that it doesn't have to be one or the other. There is a possibility of getting somewhere in-between. Now he's gotten there: somewhere in between. He has gone back to school and he and I are both working at the same mental health agency.

And we just started with a simple, "OK, can you make eye contact with me? If you can talk to me, then you can talk to other people."

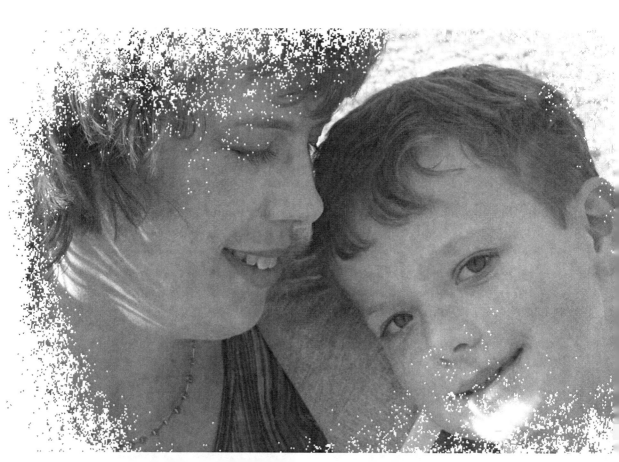

I bet everybody wishes they had a counselor like you.

I don't know about that, but I enjoy it.

What is your calling or life path? How is mental health a part of your calling?

I think that my calling in life is to reach out, get to know, and value the outcasts in society; the people who are marginalized; the people who other people just don't think about or might judge. I feel my life's calling is to really be there for people who don't have other people in their cheering section, and to give them hope, love and care. I get the same back when I give it.

"OK, can you make eye contact with me? If you can talk to me, then you can talk to other people."

When I was growing up, I always knew I was going to be a teacher. My parents were teachers and I was going to become a teacher, too. It was a given. But after my hospitalization, the education department at the University of Virginia said, "Thanks, but no thanks." They didn't want me back.

There I was: fresh out of the hospital, scared to death, not knowing what to do. I started trying to regroup. *Who am I? Where am I going in life?* I remembered back to a passage of Scripture that says, God comforts us in our struggles so that we're able to comfort others in their struggles. That passage gave direction to my life. I began to believe that maybe my mental health struggles were not for naught. I decided to pursue a major in psychology.

God gave me a specific group of people to care about: people who struggle with mental health issues. I can connect with them because of my own time in the fire. I've been there and I can really empathize with where they are. I can truly love them and care about them. God has used my experiences to work in me patience, understanding, compassion, and genuine care for people whom I wouldn't even have known existed before. He's given me a desire to advocate for the disenfranchised.

I've found that people who gave me grace rather than judgment ultimately made the biggest difference in my life. Now I want to be one of those people for others.

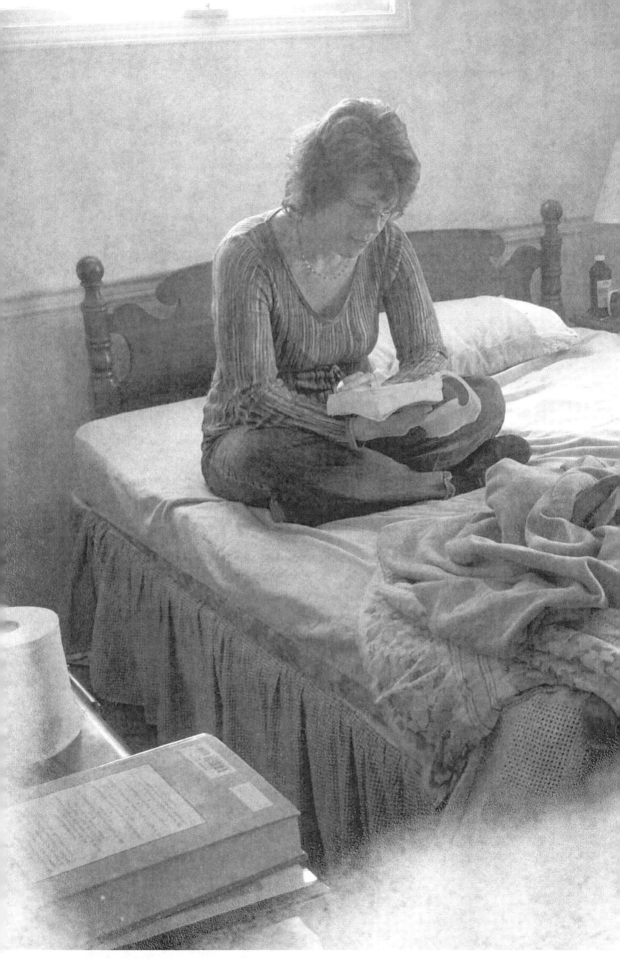

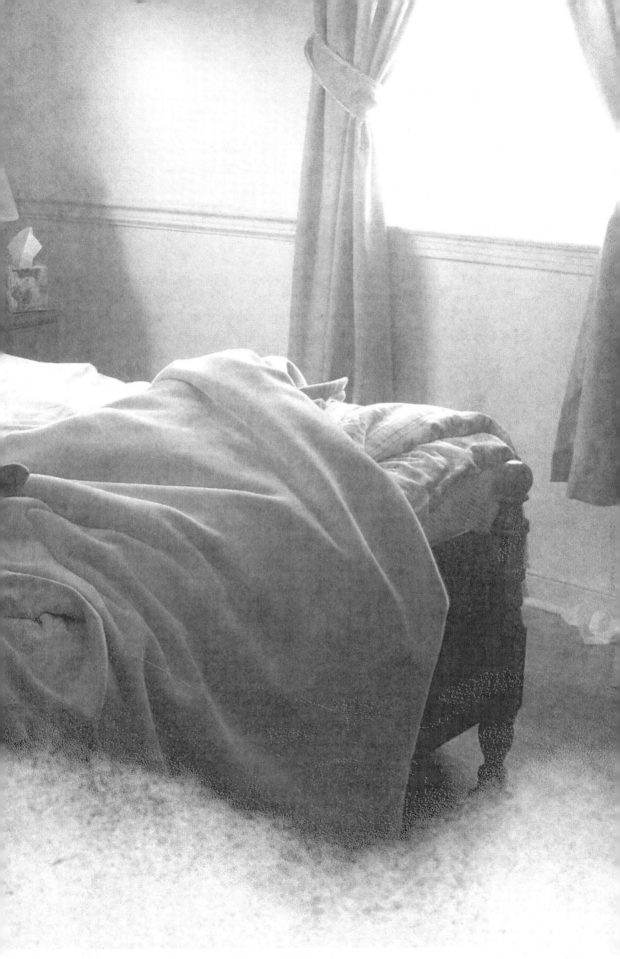

That's beautiful. Can you remember a time when you came to realize that was your calling?

When I first started working at Blue Ridge House, there was a point when I realized that the people I wanted to work with were the ones whom other people didn't want to work with. I realized that those were the people I genuinely like. I feel like one of them. I always wondered what psychiatrists and staff said about me when I wasn't there. I always thought I was the "problem patient" or the one nobody liked.

There was a time when my case load was mostly people who had been diagnosed with borderline personality disorder. Those are people some staff say they find it difficult to work with; and I just realized that I was loving it because I was really bonding and developing relationships with people. I was seeing changes.

Some of the strongest people I've ever met are members at Blue Ridge House. They've come through some major adversity and are still standing, still moving forward. There are three people in particular – one of whom is Myra, who is also in the *Firewalkers* book. I saw all three of them start out in the midst of their illness – unable to reach out or do anything. That's how I've been at some of the earlier parts of my life. Now they have moved forward and become inspirations. They've been hired as staff members in our mental health agency. Just to see them transformed from a shell trapped by their illness, to becoming free of the label – that's inspired me to look at my own symptoms differently. As I've helped them develop strategies, I found I could often use those strategies for myself.

I'm really grateful to have had the opportunity to interact with people and to give them the kind of acceptance I've needed at so many points in my own life. My experiences have blessed me by allowing my life to become intertwined with so many other lives. I think being intricately involved in other people's lives is what adds richness and depth to our existence.

I don't think much of the world appreciates the intensity of the internal struggle associated with mental illness – the way that it can destroy relationships, vocational success, hopes, dreams. Being able to come through this with a realization that life isn't over, that there are still things worth living and fighting for, requires incredible resilience. It's a resilience that you wouldn't know you had unless you found that you could indeed make it through the fire.

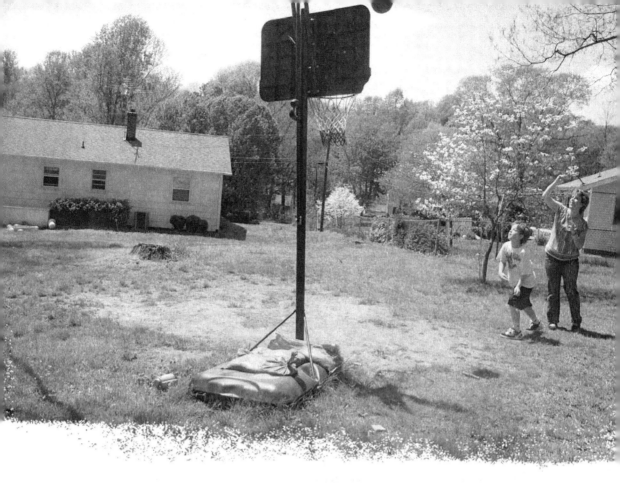

There are so many people who are "Firewalkers." I am privileged to be chosen for this book, but I think I'm representative of a lot of people who have walked through the fire of mental illness and are coming out better on the other side, coming out with purpose to their life.

Back when I was in and out of the hospital,
my dreams of getting married were shattered.
I didn't think I'd ever meet someone who'd have me.
I thought I was too broken, too messed up.

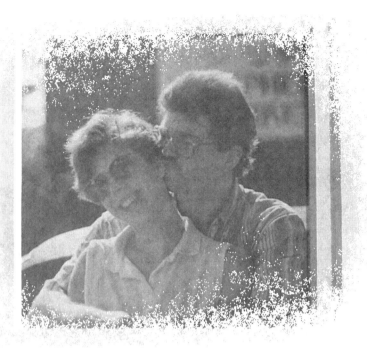

How has your experience with mental health issues affected your family life?

I met my wonderful husband at the program where I work. If I hadn't been through mental health struggles, we never would have met. Back when I was in and out of the hospital, my dreams of getting married were shattered. I didn't think I'd ever meet someone who'd have me. I thought I was too broken, too messed up. I'm hoping people who are struggling with mental health issues can look at this book and say, "Well, she's been going through this and she's still married." There's still a possibility of life beyond what you're seeing today. You don't have to give up on your dreams.

If I'm suicidal, it's especially difficult for my husband. He's thinking: "You have this wonderful life with me and the kids. Why would you want to hurt yourself?" He's worked hard at it and gotten so much better. I think now he has a sense that I just need to be heard and to know that he is there for me.

My parents have never looked up facts about mental illness – some people would say that they're in denial – but I think it's been helpful that they want to relate to me as their daughter, not as my diagnosis. I remember my dad crying the first time I went into the hospital, and yet he sent me letters while I was there, just letting me know he loved me and that he was trying to understand.

I appreciate what you said about your husband coming to understand self-destructive behavior. You've talked a little bit about cutting. Does that mean you were cutting yourself?

I was cutting myself and burning myself. This is something that's hard for people to understand, but it was a coping mechanism... I don't want to encourage anyone to do it.

I was so messed up and I cut myself to punish myself. That's what I used to stop the world and get refocused. When I was in school it felt like sometimes I couldn't figure out what I needed to do next; everything was so confusing and I didn't know what was going on in the world. It got better when I got out of school and I could refocus around work and something purposeful. This experience has helped me to understand some of the people I work with now.

What do you understand about cutting that some of your colleagues might not see?

It's not a suicidal gesture. It very seldom is. And there's a reason that people do it.

You can't just tell people to stop because it's serving a function. You need to help them find something else that will serve that same function and is healthier, rather than just shaming them or telling them it's bad. They're doing it because it's meeting a need. They're in a desperate place. It's important to be able to understand that desperation, and to then be able to talk to people about using other strategies. You have to talk about how it's a strategy that just isn't a very good one. You shouldn't get freaked out, because sometimes getting freaked out can make someone feel worse and cut more, or it can make someone feel special. So just walk in and talk to them about it.

How would your life be different if you hadn't walked your particular path?

My experience with mental illness has transformed my whole life; it's transformed how I relate; it's transformed how my boys look at the world. I grew up in a household of perfectionists. I was a very critical, judgmental person.

Now I have trouble even judging criminals – which is maybe kind of crazy – but I think you've got to meet people where they are, and see where they're coming from. My basic belief is that people want to be liked, people want to do well. I've developed an appreciation for getting to know people, getting to understand what their world is like, and not assuming that they are interacting with the world in the same way I am.

What I look for in the world has changed. I've come to realize that you don't have to be perfect to be OK. I've learned to appreciate the times when I'm not in the depths of depression – even if my house is still a mess.

Going through mental health turbulence led you to raise your kids in a different way?

I don't push them as hard to excel. Not that I don't want them to excel, but I just don't want to make them stressed out about everything in life. I want them to enjoy life. It's not that I don't want them to keep their room clean... I just haven't figured it all out yet. It's more important for me to get them out playing and doing stuff. Life has a way of not going in a straight line. Even if they get good grades, if God has a different plan for them, it's not going to matter. I care about how they feel about themselves and how they relate to other people. I've started thinking that those kind of things are more important.

My boys are seven and ten now. As they get older and into their teenage years, I want to be a mom that they can come to and talk with about their struggles. I want to raise boys who are emotionally healthy, so that even if they sometimes face a mental health struggle, they will feel comfortable getting help and doing what they need to do to move towards their own goals.

Something you've said that I really loved was, "The more fire you go through the shinier you end up on the other side." Can you tell me how that's been true for you?

When silver is burned in fire, the yucky stuff comes off. If it wasn't being burned, all that stuff would stay on. I try to think of that in the midst of the fire and hard times: God's getting the yucky stuff off of me, enabling me to be more compassionate towards other people, more caring, more humble through the fire.

I'm definitely a stronger person as a result of the firewalk I've taken over the past 20 years. If I hadn't been so desperate, if I hadn't been so needy, if I hadn't felt so alone and confused, I wouldn't have the faith that I have now. One of the things I've come to understand as a result of my mental health struggles is that the very things we'd most want to avoid in life — the most painful things — are the things that refine us and make us stronger. I believe that suffering produces perseverance, which produces character, which produces hope.

I think that my calling in life
is to reach out, get to know,
and value the **outcasts** in society;

the people who are marginalized;
the people whom other people just
don't think about or might judge.

I feel my life's calling is to really be
there for people who don't have
other people in their cheering section,
and to give them hope, love and care.

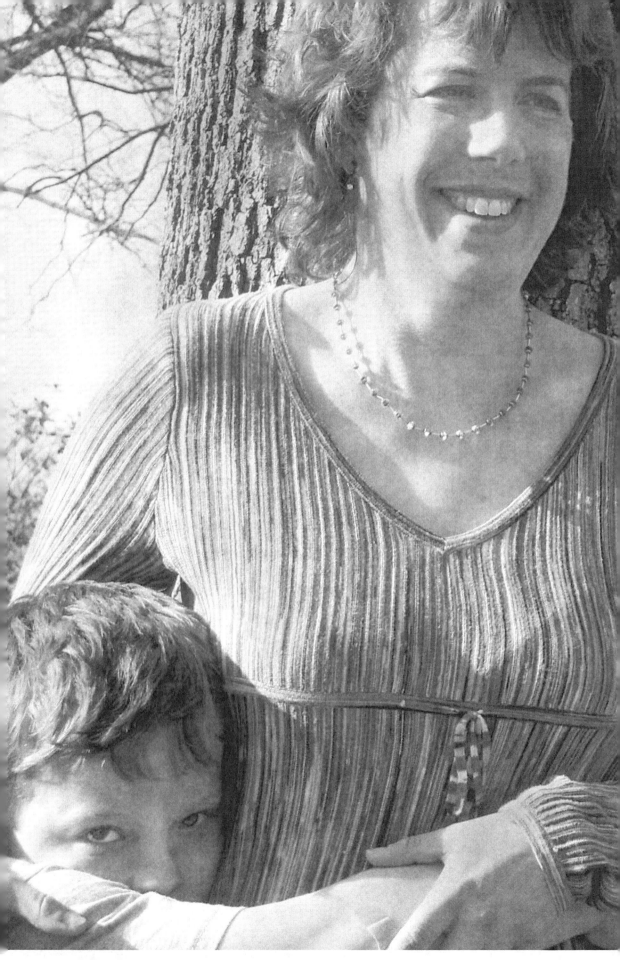

I had

a steady job at our mental health agency for more than 16 years when I decided to take a step that I hoped would move me forward in my recovery. In January 2008, after months of being "stable" but feeling depressed and unmotivated, I talked with my doctor: Was this as good as it was going to get? I wanted more. I wanted to be happy and energized in life, not just stable. However, in the ensuing months I would find out that psychiatric stability wasn't something to be taken for granted.

My psychiatrist and I agreed that I would go off the medication I was on and go into a clinical trial. I did everything the way I would counsel anyone else to do it: I followed my doctor's instructions for going off the medications exactly. I told my supervisor at work what my plans were. I asked for support during the time of being off medication. Unfortunately, I didn't do well enough off of medication to be able to get into the clinical trial.

I was like this little ticking time bomb every day. My symptoms got so bad and I began to feel so suicidal that I ended up needing to go back on medication immediately. Throughout the next few months, as I was working to get stable on medication again, I was paranoid, obsessive, and self-destructive. I kept up with my job responsibilities, and I don't think that clients could ever tell, but sometimes I would go into the chart room and cry and get very shaky.

My previous boss used to say great things about me, and the clients would say nice things, too. So when I had a relapse, I was able to feel safe and secure in getting better. My last boss weathered a lot of little storms with me, and she would always say, "You're still worthwhile. We're not going to let you go. We're not going to fire you." I didn't know until recently what a difference that makes as far as recovery goes.

During this relapse, I had a new supervisor. She is without a doubt one of the nicest people I've ever met, but when I started having mental health problems, she would throw up her hands and say, "I don't know what to do with you. I don't know what's wrong with you."

My supervisors were very frank about the fact that they didn't know how to deal with me and they just wanted me to get it back together... quickly. That was my desire as well. I saw my psychiatrist frequently. I saw my counselor weekly.

I called emergency services fairly often. I used all the tools I had accumulated over the years. However, it just wasn't to be. It was a scary time, because I couldn't "pull it together." I just didn't have the ability to rein it in.

Eventually I recovered and reached a better place mentally, emotionally, and spiritually than I had been in a long time. Unfortunately, though, there was a price to pay for taking over four months to get stable. I ended up needing to resign from my job before I got fired. It was a job that I loved, a job where I felt I was able to give back to others who were struggling in the same way I'd struggled for so much of my life.

Giving up that job was difficult. I had thought I was in an environment where I was valued for who I was and for the contributions I'd made to the agency over the years. I thought I was worth enough that supervisors would be willing to weather a mental health crisis for me. Through this situation, I was reminded just how hard it is for people (even mental health professionals) to deal with people who are actively struggling with mental health problems.

Symptoms generally aren't attractive or pleasant to deal with. They can make it hard to be around a person. It takes a firm commitment to the person and much grace to continue to be supportive in the midst of the struggle, when you may feel like you don't even like the person anymore.

I am much happier today. I am working at a local agency that provides therapy to children and families who are in difficult situations. The position seems perfectly suited to me, and my new supervisor is wonderful. She has shown me tremendous grace and has taught me so much. The agency shares many of my key values – including treating people as individuals rather than as labels, and focusing on strengths rather than on deficits. This new position has allowed me to grow in ways I couldn't have if I'd stayed in a job that had become too comfortable. I am truly blessed, and I'm able to see that daily.

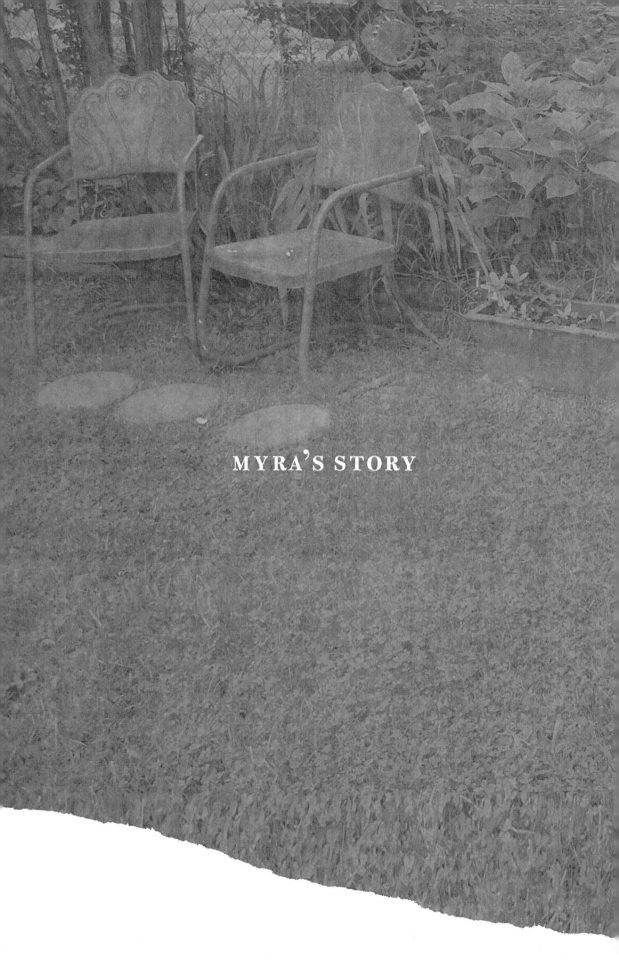

MYRA'S STORY

My life has been like a fiery furnace for over 15 years.

I have yet to meet another person whose experience has been quite like mine. I was hospitalized in psychiatric hospitals over 100 times. I was told by professionals that there was no hope for me. I was told that I would never be able to function outside of the hospital,

BUT I MANAGED TO PROVE THEM WRONG.

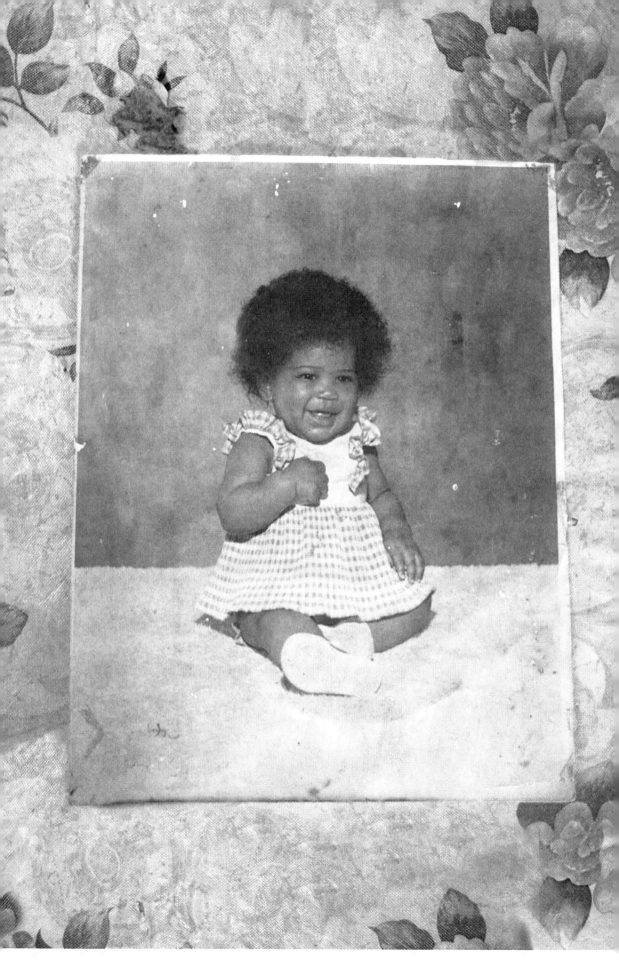

The turning

point for me wasn't one magical moment. It was a gradual thing and it had a lot to do with me involving myself with peers, involving myself with the mental health advocacy movement, and doing what I could to help myself. The realization came when I saw that I had a role to play in what was happening to me. I like the things that I'm doing right now, and I hope that greater opportunities come my way.

As poet Langston Hughes once wrote, "Life for me ain't been no crystal stair." My journey has had splinters, tacks, and boards torn up. This is a journey from oppression to liberation, from victim to survivor, and from bondage to freedom. This is a journey of hope – hope for anyone who has ever been diagnosed with a serious mental illness. I write these words for everyone who has struggled with childhood trauma, neglect, abuse, molestations, self-injurious behaviors, and suicide attempts, and for anyone who has been robbed of their livelihood. There is hope. My journey is evidence. This is my story.

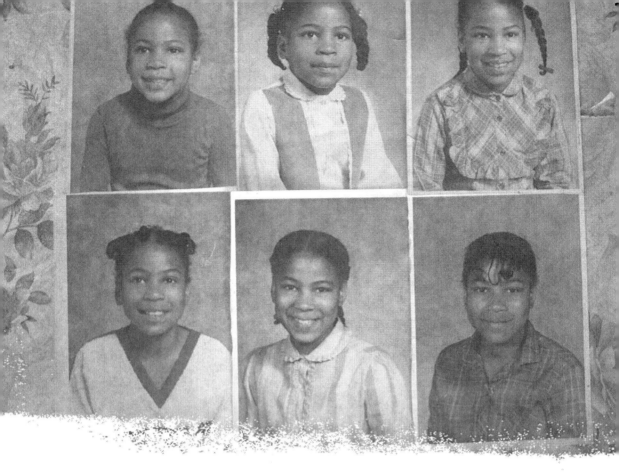

Interviews by Cynthia Power, Mitzi Ware & Debra Knighton; Photographs by Cassandra Nudel

Myra, how does your story begin?

I've always known from as early as I can remember that I was different. I didn't know what obsession meant at that time, I just knew that I stayed on things for a long time. On the last day of school I would have a major breakdown. I couldn't bear the thought of leaving my teacher.

As a child, I looked at people who lived in public housing and I thought: *Damn, they have it good. They have a kitchen they can cook in. They have indoor plumbing. They have a bathroom they can go to.* Right before the onset of my mental health problems, my family was living in real poverty.

I had my first psychiatric hospitalization when I was 12 years old, after I made some comments about suicide. I remember my parents walking me down the children's unit. I began pleading, sobbing uncontrollably. The nurse showed me my bedroom and told me that I was to make my bed every day, shower every day, and take any medication they would give me. She told me that if I didn't, they had another room waiting for me, where I would be tied down to a bed. I began to cry. The man who had hurt me was in jail, but I felt like I was in jail, too.

What I learned from my first hospitalization was this: In order to get out, you have to hide how you truly feel. You lie until you don't even feel real anymore. You learn to play the game. You smile and take your medication, and tell the staff how much better you feel, when deep inside you still feel like dying. Every morning you get dressed, make your bed, and talk therapeutic jargon all day long.

I spent all of my teen years and most of my twenties in psychiatric hospitals. The hospitals were like a dumping ground for troubled kids. There I was: a post-traumatic, majorly depressed cutter, medium to high suicide risk, with borderline and dissociative tendencies, who loved rap music, wrote poetry that didn't make sense to anyone, and dreamed of becoming an anchor for the evening news.

At age 15, I was in a hospital where the staff restrained me. They were very abusive. I can't begin to tell you how traumatizing this is for someone who has been violated in the past. Every time and I felt myself being physically held down by strong men, I was reliving the assault. In my mind, I was being violated over and over again. I made a promise to myself that when I turned 18, I would seek legal help to address these issues. I stayed true to that promise, and my case became a class action lawsuit, which was settled out of court.

When I was 18 years old a doctor said to me, "We're going to get you set up in a group home." I remember thinking: *There has to be more for me than this. This isn't the end for me.* While he was busy making arrangements for placement visits, I hit the books and, in less than a month, I had obtained my high school equivalency diploma, taken the SATs, and filled out college applications. When it came time for me to go to a placement visit I said, "I have a different plan for my life and I think I'm going to go to Virginia Commonwealth University instead and see how I do there."

In order to get out, you have to hide how you truly feel.

...You smile and take your medication, and tell the staff how much better you feel, when deep inside you still feel like dying.

My late teens and early twenties were like when the levees broke in New Orleans and the water came in. Everything was all over the place – nothing but pure chaos. Through all this, I still didn't think there was anything wrong with me. I always had a reason to blame somebody else. I didn't realize that I had a major role to play in my recovery.

Then one day I read this book about mental health diagnosis and the first thing I said to myself was, *Oh my God! This is what's wrong with me!* It was devastating, but it was almost a relief. It was like holding a mirror up to myself and looking at it – there was all the wrecking relationships, all the suicide attempts, all the legal charges and loss of employment, everything that I had ever experienced.

Can you tell us more about what your daily life was like when you were at your lowest point?

Well, it was actually quite a simple life because most of my time was spent sleeping. There's 24 hours in a day. I would spend about 18 hours sleeping. For about six months I couldn't get out of bed. I wasn't showering, I wasn't doing anything. I would get up once a day when my mom had cooked dinner and I would eat and go right back to bed. I remember the despair of her saying, "Why don't you come and help me out in the kitchen?" and I would go down there and try to do one thing and I would just end up back in my room because it just seemed too overwhelming for me.

There is a saying, "Where there is no hope there is no light." The point that I began to have hope is when things began to turn around for me.

I always had a reason to blame somebody else.

I didn't realize that I had a major role to play in my recovery.

It seems like coming to the realization that you had some responsibility in your mental health recovery and that you couldn't just depend on the hospital and the system was a major step.

I was addicted to going in and out of hospitals. I spent a lot of time looking for somebody to fix me. All I had to do was exist; they took care of everything else. In my early twenties, I researched the best psychiatric hospitals in America. One of them was Johns Hopkins University in Maryland... so I up and moved there. Then I researched Duke University and moved down to Durham, North Carolina. Every time I was expecting the same thing and every time I was not yielding very good results.

I spent so much time in hospitals. As sick as it might sound, there was something very comforting about other people saying, "We'll take care of you. We'll make it better." At one of the hospitals, there was a nurse named Robin. She'd known me since I was 14 years old, and she had zero tolerance for my antics. One time when they had called security on me she said, "Myra, you're too smart for all of this. You're either going to go through life continuing to go in and out of hospitals, or you're going to do something with yourself." She looked down at her watch and said, "You have two minutes to decide." Security was on their way.

I broke down and told her, "I want to have a better life. I want more for my life." And she sent security away. We had a heart-to-heart talk. I thought about it more and more and more and wondered: *Is this is going to be my life, going in and out of hospitals, never knowing when the police are going to show up at my door? Is this the story I'm going to have to tell my whole life?*

Robin was the first person in my life who really challenged me. She had only seen me at my worst because the only time she saw me was when I was in the hospital, but she knew enough to believe that I could be more. That day was the first time I had the thought that I could do something. I didn't know what I could do, but I thought: *Maybe there is something else for me besides constantly going in and out, in and out, in and out of the hospital. Maybe this doesn't have to be my life.*

Then in 2002 I had a roommate who committed suicide at the hospital. When you're in the hospital, you become quite close with your roommate fairly quickly. I identified with this person so much; I liked this person so much. If I didn't change something, I would be next. After that, I knew that I had to get myself out of the hospital – quick, fast, and in a hurry. It was a challenge because I didn't have any tools at the time. I didn't know anything about mental health recovery. All I had was a very good therapist. But I knew I had to keep myself out of the hospital.

The smartest thing I did was join the Advisory Council at my mental health agency. The Council is made up of people who receive services at our agency. I can't say I joined because I wanted to further Council objectives. I didn't even know what the Council was. Somebody told me that they had great food at their meetings, so I went.

At the meeting I met an amazing man named Paul Patrick. I asked him how long he had been out of the hospital, and he said ten years. I remember thinking *Ten years!! How is that possible? What are these people doing that I'm not doing? I can't seem to stay out for a month!*

That's when things started to work in my life. It wasn't the medication; it wasn't the treatment; it wasn't going to the best psychiatrist in town. It was being connected with other people who had been in the mental health system — people who had walked that walk and had advice to give me.

I can't say that something magically happened to me one day and I thought, *Oh, I understand everything about mental health recovery.* It was gradual. I began to learn about other opportunities. I went to a leadership academy for people in the mental health system, I took a recovery class, I went to meetings of mental health advocates, and all the while time was building up out of the hospital.

Even though I had my own problems, the Advisory Council was about business. All the energy that I had been focusing into making chaos in my own life, I now focused into planning conferences. One day, I looked back and realized, *You know, I don't need to go into the hospital.*

What's your hope in telling your story?

I always felt bad about the trauma I experienced as a child, but there was a point in my early twenties where my counselor told me about a 12-year-old girl whose father had abused her. She was getting ready to go to court and she was terrified. My counselor asked me if I would talk to the girl. I said, "Me?! What am I going to say to her?" and she replied, "Well, she wants to know what's going to happen in court and what your experience was." So I talked to the girl and relieved all her worries and my counselor said, "Wow, you did an amazing job."

For the first time in my life, I felt like maybe what I had gone through wasn't without a reason. Maybe it was meant for me to tell this girl this, to lighten her load. That was a point where I really felt like I was learning to play the hand I was dealt.

For the first time in my life, I felt like maybe what I had gone through wasn't without a reason.

If I can continue in the mental health advocacy movement, pushing forward and making things better for the next person, then it's all going to be worth it. I look at it like this: we're only on this earth for a little bit of time. This book may be around when we're not here anymore.

If I can use my experience to make the load lighter for the person coming behind me, then it's well worth it. I hope that people can look at my story and see what I've been through and maybe they won't make as many mistakes as I did. I've already been there and I've made enough mistakes for me and 100 other people.

Tell us a story about when you were in the fire.

I experienced abuse as a child. I went to court and had the person sentenced to 25 years in jail. In my adulthood he was released from jail early and I saw him in a store. It brought back a lot of bad memories and sent me into a downward momentum.

I was a walking time bomb. Very quickly I became self-destructive. I wasn't sleeping well and I was having a lot of nightmares and I was unsure about going out. I would be on Interstate 64 driving 95 miles per hour and hoping I would wreck. It's sad that not only did I not respect myself, but I didn't even respect anybody else that was on the road.

The "fire" and the low point came when one night I took a combination of Vicodin and Ativan and chased it with a bottle of vodka. I woke up three days later in the intensive care unit. I pleaded with God that since he wanted me to live, he would have to show me how to live.

How were you able to move from seeing yourself as a victim to seeing yourself as a survivor?

I had been letting the abuser control my life and have a lot of power. That's something I was doing to myself. It was one thing to be victimized, but I was letting myself be further victimized by not moving on. I didn't feel like I had

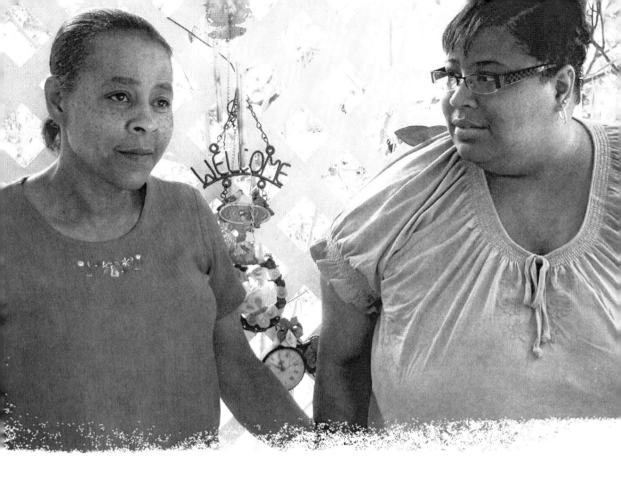

any power in the situation. I found an online sanctuary where people who have experienced childhood trauma posted their poems and stories. I realized I looked at myself as still being a victim, when I should have looked at myself as a survivor, because I survived the whole atrocity.

What is your experience coming from an African American community?

When I let my faith community know that I was in the psychiatric hospital, they came and stood by my side. They would visit me, pray with me, and bring me the items that I would request. I think this has to do with the history of the black church. Through the civil rights movement, the church was the center of social and human services for black people. When people haven't had any-where else to turn, the church has always been there for them.

As an African-American, I didn't live through the civil rights movement, but it's my history. Martin Luther King Jr. wasn't here to see his dream of black people and white people sitting together in harmony, but it did come true. I know that if we're going to make things better, we have to make choices now to affect the people of tomorrow.

Now I am the chair of our mental health advisory council, and we do a lot of letter writing voicing our opinion to politicians and visiting the legislators. If we're going to affect policy and make things better for the people coming after us, that's something that we need to act on today.

I come from a history of people that have been oppressed and were able to rise above. In my mind, I come from greatness and that's what I expect from myself: greatness. Slaves were oppressed, but they still sang songs and hymns. There was this inner joy that no one could take away. I felt like I was oppressed having a psychiatric diagnosis, living in poverty, and coming from a family that had domestic violence early on. But everything that was pushing me down still couldn't take away my joy.

What part of your recovery do you feel most proud of?

I remember my parents coming to my graduation when I became a Certified Mental Health Peer Support Specialist. In the whole time that I've been ill, my parents have had very little to celebrate. So this was a very big day and all my family was there and I had a chance to stand up and to talk a little bit about my experience and to thank people. If you could have seen how proud my mother was that day. She brought me flowers.

At the graduation ceremony, I was thinking: *Everything that I've been through, it's all come to this point right here and this is the point where I take my life back. There is a different direction for me now and greater things are going to happen to me if I stay along this path.* It was the first time in my life that I was able to see that my mental health struggles weren't in vain; there was a plan and a purpose.

Have there been people who helped lighten the load for you?

The beauty of my family is that they never treated me any differently. They treated me like they would treat somebody in the hospital for a physical condition – not something to be ashamed of. My grandmother had unconditional love for me, no matter what I did. She saw nothing but good in me and that helped bring me to the other side. My parents also support anything I do.

I've been seeing the same therapist for the last eight years and we've just recently got to the point where she can challenge me on things, and I don't become emotionally unstable. Now we're having the type of therapy that should have been happening from the start. I asked her once, "If you would have known

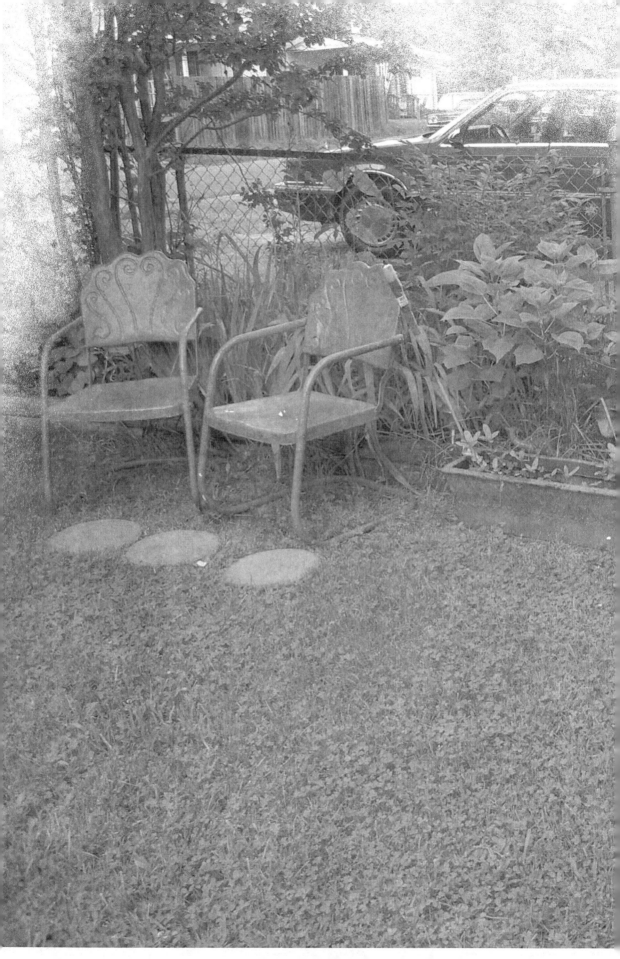

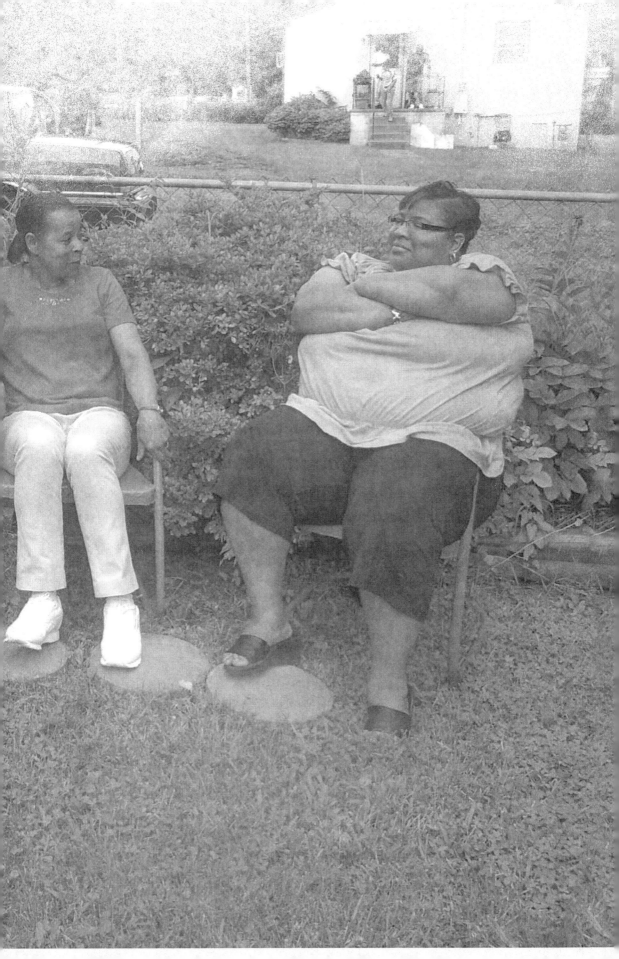

that all this trouble was coming in your door the first time you met me, would you have seen me anyway, and continued to see me?" She just kind of chuckled and said, "Well Myra, I'm still here."

I also want to talk about Debra, who is in this *Firewalkers* book. When I met Debra, I was going to the mental health day program where she works. I felt like I didn't fit in, so I would just sit and do nothing all day. Every day she came up to me and invited me to do things. Every day I said no. But it didn't stop her. She kept inviting me. Finally I thought, *Let me just go to one thing to get this lady off my back.* I ended up going to Debra's group on Current Issues in Mental Health. It was very powerful.

There were times when all the other staff wrote me off. Debra was the one person who held out hope for me. No matter where I was, she saw something in me that nobody else saw. She saw it; she nurtured it; she gave me hope when I didn't have hope for myself.

Now when I see someone walking down the street talking to himself, my first thought is: He might be having a difficult time with his illness.

What is your dream or hope? What is your next step?

My dream is that I would get to the point where I know I have a mental health diagnosis, but it wouldn't be something I have to think about a lot during the day. I would like for mental illness to be a smaller part of who I am and other aspects of myself to shine through and be a bigger part.

Most of my friends and most of my activities relate to mental health. I've been really making the effort lately to try to meet other people. I joined a new church. I just got a scholarship to take classes at our local community college. I'm very excited about learning new things. I joined the gym and I instantly found a friend, and our connection doesn't have anything to do with mental health.

I'm just beginning to see that there is a life outside of having a mental health diagnosis. There is a big world out there. When you have a diagnosis, your life can revolve around that — talking to the case manager, talking to the doctor, talking to the therapist, taking medication, making sure you do all these things they've instructed you to do. Sometimes it's easy to forget that there is a big world out there, a world full of so many different opportunities.

I really feel like I'm just beginning to enjoy life. I just started to plan a vacation and it's the first time I can remember that I've ever taken a vacation. My friend and I were talking and we said, "You know, we spent so much time running in and out of the hospital that we didn't really get a good chance to enjoy life". Right now we're just doing something that everyday people do all the time: taking a vacation.

I'm very excited right now about enjoying simple things. I like to sit outside at night and watch people. Somebody will pass by with a baby and the baby may look up and smile. That's something very simple, but there was a time when I couldn't enjoy those things.

I would also like to have a family; I would like to have a husband and a child. I would like to eventually work full-time and get completely off of benefits. I would like to return to school and finish my degree. I'd like to write a book. Writing has gotten me through the fire, through the dark, through the rain, through everything.

What have you seen or understood about life as a result of your mental health journey? What have you experienced that you wouldn't have experienced otherwise?

My life has played out the way it has for a reason. I'm walking this path and opportunities are coming my way leading to bigger things. If I had never encountered mental illness, I wouldn't be working as a peer support specialist now, I wouldn't have sat on the Board of Directors of my mental health agency, and I wouldn't be involved with our advisory council. I wouldn't have the same compassion. Now when I see someone walking down the street talking to himself, my first thought is: *He might be having a difficult time with his illness.*

Going through mental health struggles has drawn me closer to God. When I didn't have anybody else that I could call on or depend on, I felt like God was there by my side and his mercy was upon me. I believe God has a plan and purpose for my life and that's still being revealed to me.

Today I am a person who sleeps quite well.

It's not that I have a lot of money in my bank account; it's not that I live in the best place or drive the best car, but I wake up every morning with anticipation:

What's going to happen today?
Thank God I'm still here and that I didn't die
the many times that I tried to take my life.

CARLA'S STORY

My life would be smaller
if I hadn't experienced
mental illness.

I probably would not see the bigger
picture of the world and the way things are.
I feel very blessed that I did walk
through the fire.

It opened my eyes to seeing humanity.

When I *was 32 years old and starting a children's theme party business, I started believing my dentist was following me.*

I thought my teeth were bugged and there were cameras installed everywhere I went. I remember the day I first thought I was being followed. I remember the first time I looked over and thought the dentist was there watching me. My whole family – my father, sister, brother, their kids – were out at an ice show. When they got home, I started acting differently. I thought the cameras were there.

My business was incorporated, I had ordered $5,000 worth of inventory, and I would be up until two in the morning taking photographs for the catalog. I was trying to keep everything perfect – the perfect house, the perfect schedule. I thought that my dentist and half the county were rooting for me to succeed; I would turn on the radio so they could give me messages. If a song came on the radio advertising a certain church, I thought that was a message for me to go to that church, so I would run from church to church.

During that beginning phase, I was euphoric. I felt like I had stepped out of the rain into this new world where everything was intense. I believed there was a good side and an evil side, and the dentist was on the good side. Then my emotions began to fluctuate rapidly. I made my husband change the locks on the door. I locked my journals in a box, but that wasn't good enough. I started burning what I wrote. I left a note for the "evil people:"

I don't want anyone else to know what I wrote in my journal.

Your purpose may have originally been all in fun, but it's not anymore.

If there is a recording device in the house it needs to be removed.

I was in psychosis for nine months before I got help. Nobody knew what was going on. Even though we had a history of mental illness in my family, it had never been talked about, so no one knew why I was acting so different. I kind of lucked into getting help: My husband and I were going to a marriage counselor and I said something that tipped her off. She immediately referred me to a psychiatrist. Wisely, the psychiatrist did not try to convince me

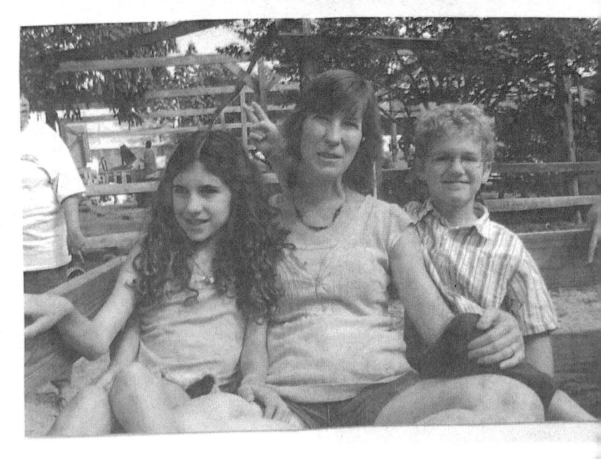

that my hallucinations were not real. He gave me some medicine and told me it would help me deal with stress. I took it.

That's when the real walking through the fire began. I went on an anti-psychotic medication and a few weeks later I realized how faulty my thinking had been. My head stopped feeling as if it were about to explode from the thoughts pouring in, but I became catatonic at work. I couldn't function. I lost my job. My creativity was gone; I was emotionally flat. I could not bathe the kids or go into stores.

I had three phases of reality: In the first phase, I couldn't concentrate on people, television, or writing. In the second phase, I couldn't tolerate anything, and I had to lie in a dark and quiet room with a pillow over my head. In the third phase, I felt a little like myself but tired and anxious about going back into phase one again. I would cycle through this many times a day.

I wasn't able to hold a conversation. I wasn't able to follow the directions on a box of macaroni and cheese. I progressed to not being able to be around people at all. It took a couple years of adjusting the dosage and medications before I began to feel better. I didn't feel like myself again - I felt better than I had before. Going through this had transformed me, spiritually and emotionally.

This is my story about how my illness developed, how I survived it, how I live with it, and how it has transformed my life.

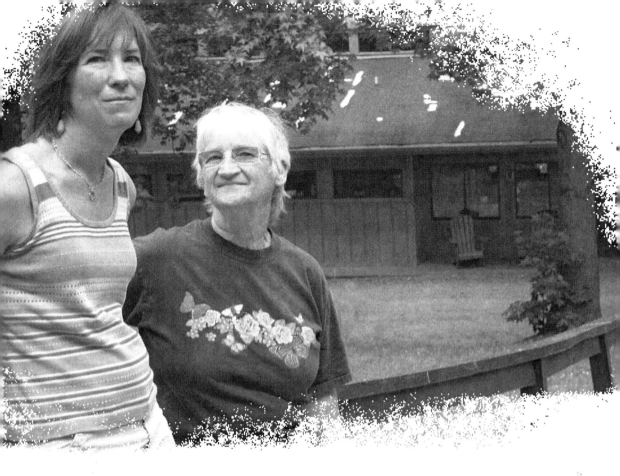

*My mom continually told me I would get better
when I didn't think I'd get better.*

*She said, "Other people have gotten better,
you will get better."*

Interviews by Cynthia Power, Debra Knighton, Bev Ball & Cassandra Nudel; Photographs by Cassandra Nudel

---

Carla, you've talked about how someone can hold the hope for you until you have it yourself. Was there somebody like that in your life, someone that held onto hope for you until you could get to that place?

That was my mom. She held hope for me when I had none for myself. When she found out what I had and how ill I was, she learned all she could about mental health. She would come over in the evenings and fix dinner because I couldn't concentrate long enough to do that. She would bathe the kids, and she would put the kids on my lap and I would rock them (I could at least do that part). Then she would put them to bed, put *me* to bed, and go home. It felt like she did that forever. She said it was actually four or five months – it felt like forever to me.

My mom continually told me I would get better when I didn't think I would. She said, "Other people have gotten better; you will get better."

I'm curious about having the challenge of going through a mental health crisis while having small children.

I really do feel like I'm a better parent because of having walked through the fire. It was a challenge during the time I was at my lowest, but we made it through together. It has improved me as a parent, and my kids have learned things that they wouldn't have learned otherwise.

The worst part was not being able to feel emotion. This is awful to say, but it's the only way I can describe it: When I held my kids, it felt like they were just a sack of potatoes on my lap. Even though I was not doing well, somewhere inside of me I knew they still needed that touch and that connection with me, so I held them and rocked them every day.

I would wake up in the morning with the thought, *How am I going to get through this day?* Fortunately, when I was at my lowest point, I had a lot of support from my mom and my husband and two neighbors. One neighbor would take my daughter to preschool and the other neighbor would watch my son. I told my neighbors I had a "nervous breakdown" because I didn't want to say "schizophrenia." Later I went back and told them I had been diagnosed with schizophrenia.

Prior to going into psychosis, my house was the one all the neighborhood kids visited to enjoy crafts, throw water balloons, and come to themed birthday parties. Now my home is once again the place for kids to hang out, have holiday parties, and enjoy birthday celebrations.

So your kids have walked through this fire with you?

Yes. They're very caring and compassionate children, *very* caring and compassionate. When my son plays soccer, he always runs and checks on other children who have fallen or may have gotten hurt. If my children are around someone with special needs or a younger child in distress, they are always quick to show empathy and to try to help. We talk a lot about how it is important to help others and about the work I do. They understand when I have to take a phone call because someone else really needs support. They know that not everyone has a mom and dad that can be there for them.

My kids and I talk about how people with psychiatric symptoms are sometimes abandoned by their families. They say, "Mom, I would never do that to you."

What happened with your marriage?

It was really, really, really hard on my husband. I mean *really* hard. I was very argumentative when I was in psychosis. I would think he was smiling a certain way as some hidden signal and I would just go into rages.

My husband worked two jobs because we had lost an income – my income. He stood by me. It was very stressful for him, but he did hang in there. He stuck around even though I was not pleasant to be around. My husband and mother took care of me and took care of my two children until I started to recover.

We've been married… it'll be 18 years this June 30th. I think our marriage is even stronger now than it was before.

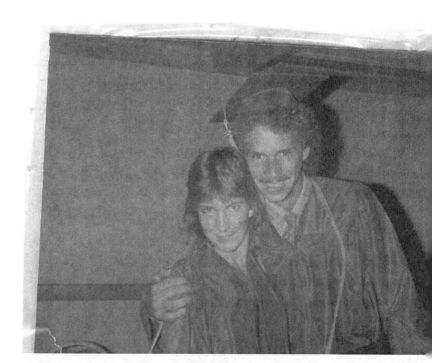

What kind of reaction did you receive from other family members?

My husband didn't tell my in-laws that I became ill. It was kept a secret because of stigma. I feared being judged. Then when somebody in my husband's family developed mental health issues, I told my father-in-law my story. I didn't expect this reaction from him, but he said, "You're a blessing to our family."

Wow.

It was the total opposite of what I was expecting.

Looking back, when was your life first impacted by mental health issues?

My first encounter with mental illness was with my brother. He was 13: wonderful, creative, artistic, loving, compassionate, and a gifted artist. He made clothes with leather-work and shark-toothed necklaces. His suicide was a great loss for the world as well as our family.

Was there a lot of talk about mental health in your family afterwards?

There was none. In my family, mental illness was something you didn't speak of. It was a hushed thing.

After my brother's suicide, my father began having delusions and paranoid thoughts. He didn't get help; he didn't get treatment; he self-medicated with alcohol. I think sometimes it might be harder for men to admit they have an illness. The stigma is so great.

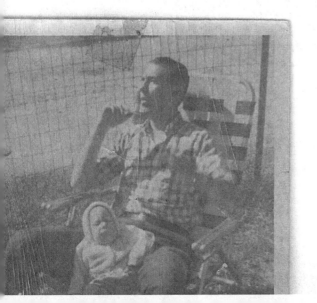

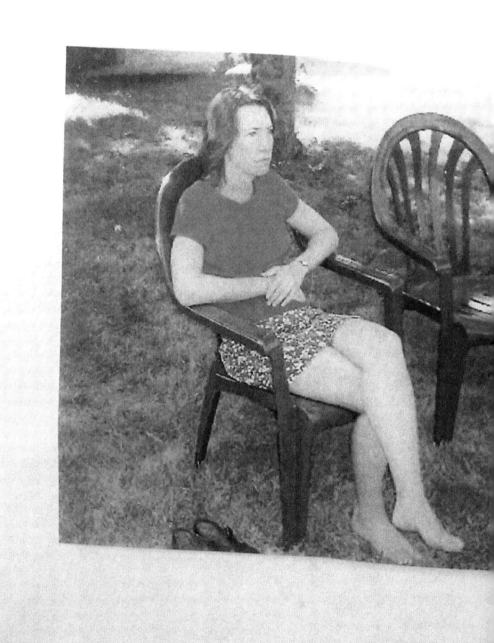

When I got older, my father would often show up on my front doorstep. I lived in the city down the street from bars. When I opened the door to go to work, he would be sitting there on my front porch with a bleeding head. I saw that he was more often a victim of violence because of his illness; he was never a perpetrator of violence. That's important for people to understand. A diagnosis of mental illness doesn't make one more likely to be violent – more often, we are the victims.

My father made numerous suicide attempts: jumping out of a moving vehicle, driving his van into a tree. We called the crisis center in Richmond, and they came to my house and told us that we needed to just admit that my father was an alcoholic. We tried to say, "No, even when he's not drinking, he's not OK. He's not doing well." But they didn't even look at the possibility that something else was wrong. We still didn't get any help for him.

When I went into psychosis at thirty-two, I really felt for my father and understood why things happened the way they had. I knew what it was like to have hallucinations and paranoid thoughts, and I knew how those things can change your behavior. I came to understand that he had no control over that.

I took care of my father the last eight months of his life. By that time, I could talk a little bit about my psychiatric diagnosis with him. My father still couldn't admit that he dealt with mental illness. That was hard to see. The quality of his life could have been so much better.

My kids and I talk about how people with mental illness are sometimes abandoned by their families. They say, "Mom, I would never do that to you."

What was the turning point in your mental health recovery?

For quite a few years I had been just living *day to day* and not really going anywhere. I thought that my life was just going to be stuck where it was, and that I didn't have meaning or purpose. I was just staying home and getting through the day.

Then my mom began teaching classes for family members of people diagnosed with mental illness, and she invited me to come to a group to share my story. Once I got up there and started talking... I realized how far I had come. I thought, "Hey! I *am* doing much better. I *did* get through that period. I *did* survive it, and I am a stronger person because of it."

That was the turning point. I decided at that moment that I wanted to work with my peers. I didn't know anything about mental health advocacy and peer support. I didn't know there was a mental health recovery movement. I had been going to a private psychiatrist through my husband's insurance. I didn't know if I'd ever met anybody else who dealt with mental illness.

So I went home and searched for trainings. That's how I became involved. I went to a mental health leadership training where I began connecting with my peers and that started to change my life. I learned about people who are uniting and trying to make improvements to mental health services, reduce stigma, and improve life for themselves and others. And I learned about VOCAL – the organization that created this *Firewalkers* book. My life started moving forward.

Today, I work as a mental health peer specialist. I facilitate mental health recovery classes. I co-founded a peer support group. I told my recovery story in the newspaper. I speak out about mental health by giving talks at conferences, psychiatric hospitals, and police stations.

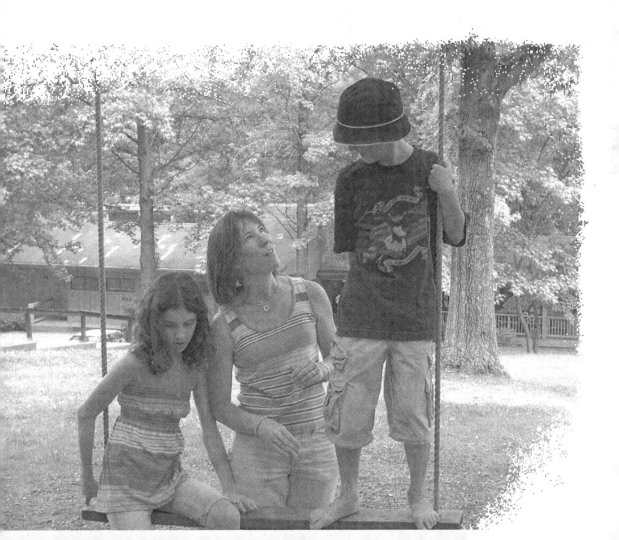

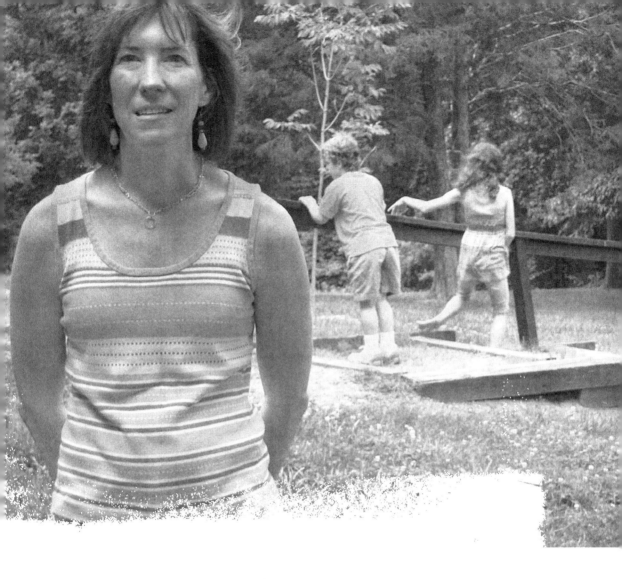

People in the mental health system are dying twenty-five years earlier than the general population.

After finding that out, I feel that
my future life path is promoting whole health care.
A real wellness center is the next step on my journey.

Have you thought about the next steps to getting there?

We're at the beginning stages of working on it: the Friends4Recovery Wellness Education and Support Center. We started the outline of a proposal, budget, and vision statement.

How do you define mental health recovery? How much of your recovery was self-motivated, and how much was impacted by others?

Recovery to me is living a full, productive, meaningful life that I direct. Getting my life back. I believe true recovery has to be self-motivated. When I was going through my darkest point I realized that nobody can recover *for* me; I have to be able to get through this. I facilitate mental health recovery groups that help people create a plan called WRAP (Wellness Recovery Action Plan). I very much believe in WRAP. Using my Plan, I've been able to catch early warning signs and escape going into psychosis again.

Have you done that on your own or with the help of other people or a combination of both?

A combination of both. The first time I didn't notice I was starting to have symptoms, my husband noticed. I was going into the nonstop chatter and I said, "I guess I'd better go to the doctor; it's been a week or so since I've slept through the night or maybe even a few weeks." He said, "It's been a few *months* since you've slept through the night. You're up every night and you're talking nonstop. You've got to do something."

The second time was when I started to go into a depression this past Christmas. It happened after a close family member went into psychosis. Seeing him brought back memories. I knew what he was going through and how terrified and out of touch with reality he felt and what he was going to have to go through to recover. I just cried at first, but then I started feeling flat. I went into a breakdown where I was unable to stop crying and unable to stop a cycle of thoughts. We had to temporarily increase some medication to get me straightened out.

I realized later that I wasn't using my WRAP plan during this period. I was just *going, going, going* until bedtime. That's when I realized how important my WRAP plan is and that I have to make time for it no matter what's going on.

What were some of the actions you took in your recovery?
From the time you were diagnosed and your world came crashing down,
what was the first thing you did?

I tried to educate myself, but at that time there weren't—and there still aren't—a lot of positive books out there to help me, definitely not a book like *Firewalkers*. I read a lot of negative things about schizophrenia. I thought, *Well this is it. You have a mental illness. This is all there is to your life now.* It was very bleak.

I wish there had been a book like *Firewalkers* available to me then. I wish I had known about peer support earlier. It's been seven years since I first got help. It took two years for me to get on the right medication and start to feel a little like myself. Then it took another three years to realize my life wasn't over and that I could move forward and have a purposeful, meaningful life.

If there had been something hopeful out there earlier, maybe my journey might have been a little quicker, but I still wouldn't change anything. I think everything had meaning.

Do you want to say any more about spirituality and how it's helped you through?

There's a reason I went through what I did. It's a spiritual reason. I remember sitting on my front porch chain smoking cigarettes. I would sit in my rocking chair and I would pray to pull through this because my kids needed me. I promised that when I came through this I would share with others that God had helped pull me through. I believe that I was meant to go down this path and I feel like it's my duty now to help others and to share how I used my faith and prayer to pull me through my darkest time.

After doing all this exploring of churches... did you ultimately find a faith community where you belonged?

When I became ill and started having the delusions, our church wasn't very supportive. They kind of wanted to wash their hands of us.

I joined a new church five years ago. At the time I didn't feel the need to tell the pastor that I had been diagnosed with a mental illness. Later I revealed it, and the pastor said that it was caused by sin. Unfortunately there are still churches out there that believe mental illness is a defect of character or it's caused by your own sin or your family's sin – that's what this pastor was saying.

I would like to find a good church. I believe there is a good church out there for me. Prior to my illness, I was full of anxiety, worry, self-doubt and questioning – always looking at the negative things that have happened in my life. Since the illness, I put more trust in God and believe that what's supposed to happen is going to happen.

How have your goals, values, and vision for your life changed as a result of your mental health journey?

When I feel hesitant now, I just think back on everything that happened and say to myself, "If you could go through that, you can get up and speak in public or "You can start a support group" or "You can start a wellness center." I say, "It may be out of your comfort zone, and you may be doing things you've never done before, but look what you've been through."

I was very shy before. I was never a person who would get up and speak in front of people. You never would have imagined that I'd turn into the person I am today. If someone had told me then that I would be in a book, I probably wouldn't have believed them.

EDITOR'S NOTE: *At time of press, Carla has just received a grant of $200,000 to create the Friends4Recovery Whole Health Center, the first and only peer-run mental health wellness center in Chesterfield County*

What I went through made me who I am today

and gave me the passion that I have

TO END THE STIGMA

and show that **people can recover** from mental illness.

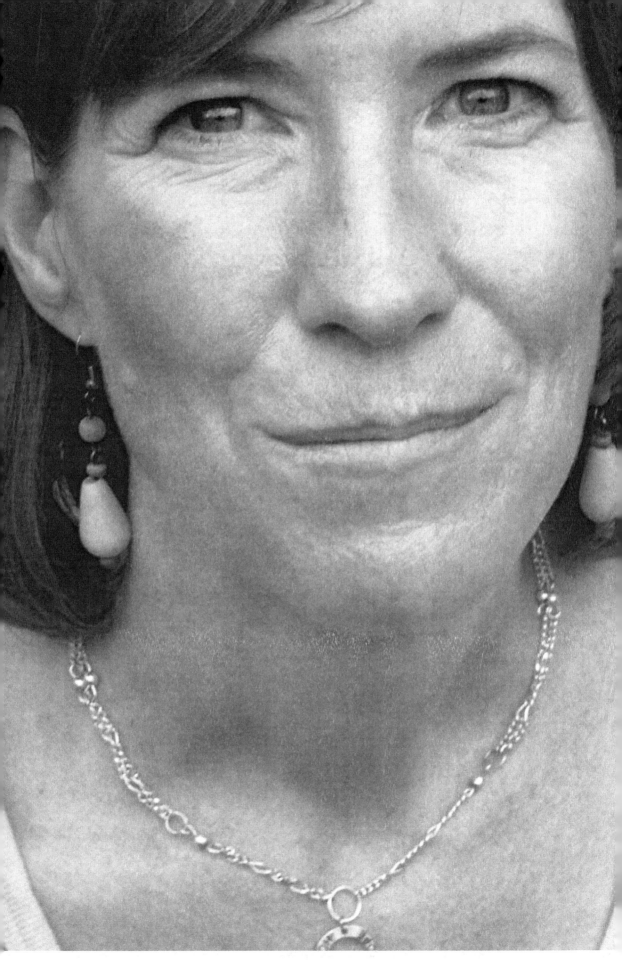

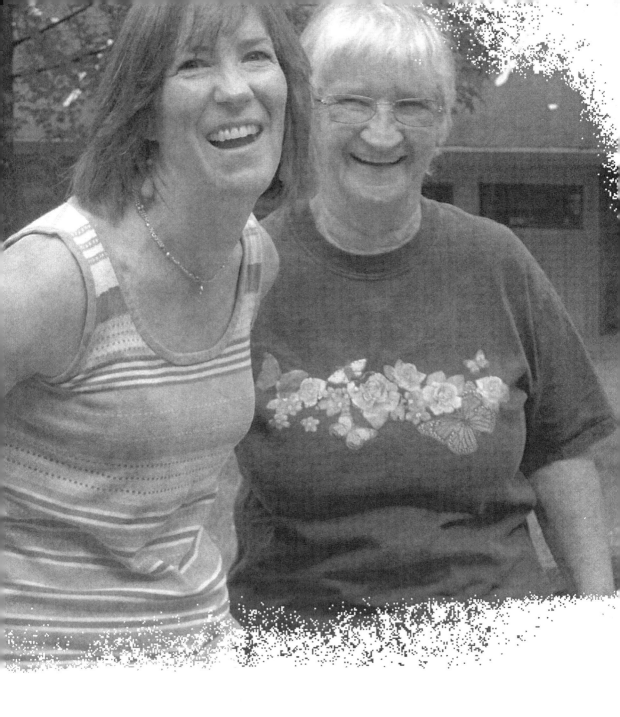

Many families can have a difficult time understanding what is happening when a loved one is experiencing a mental health crisis. How do you see what happened with Carla?

Carla came back to be more of herself – more whole, more outgoing, more determined, and much stronger than before.

When Carla was going through her hardest time, what was it that you did that you felt made the greatest difference?

I was a sounding board. Carla made the decisions. I encouraged her and helped her find things. I listened.

You were an amazing support for Carla. Not everyone has that experience. Some people feel their families are an obstacle or contribute to the problem. How did you come to have the ability to do it differently?

I had dealt with mental illness in the past and not done as well. My son Michael died by suicide at age 13 – never having been diagnosed. Then when my first husband became ill, he developed fixated ideas, and we were never able to resolve the issues. So this time with Carla, I learned more about the illness and I had family support. That made a big difference.

You have to believe that people who are ill are going to get well. And you have to be supportive along the way, so the family doesn't lose everybody. A lot of families go through a negative phase. People get stuck in that place; families become divided. There's a lot of blaming and misunderstanding. If you don't work through that, you can't be supportive.

There's no reason people can't have their full lives back. Carla has that and even more.

JONI'S STORY

One gorgeous day I am driving on this country road, just for the drive in Washington State. It is like the yellow brick road, winding with all these little houses and gardens. I am awed and happy. I see an elder woman in her garden wearing a sun hat and I stop to say, *"I'm lost. Can you tell me how to get out of here?"* She says, *"No, dear. I'm sorry. I don't know how."*

When she tells me she can't help me find my way out, I become paralyzed. I feel like I want to hurt this woman. I want to shake her and yell, *"Tell me how to get out of here!"*

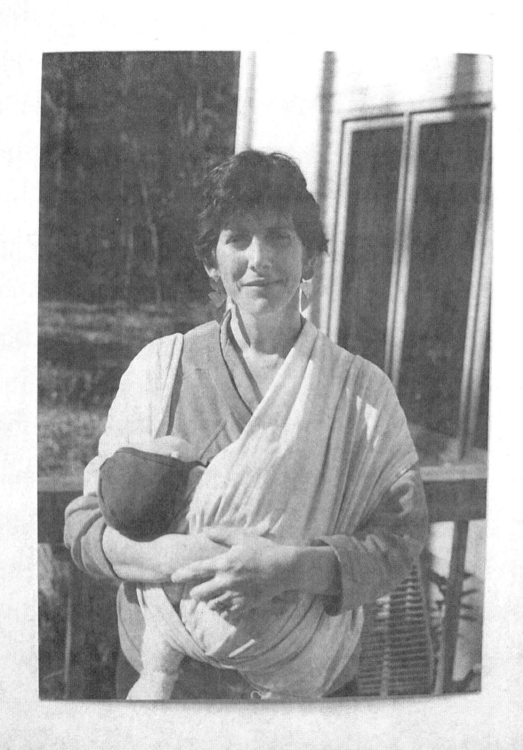

I cling

to the door of my car with all that I have and I get it on the spot: "I **do** have a problem. It's not normal to want to kill someone because they can't give you directions." I hold onto my car until it passes, and I drive away and drive right to the mental health clinic.

I show up at the clinic unexpectedly. I'd been there once before, but the psychiatrist told me to wait three weeks before getting treatment because he was going on vacation. This time, I demand to see someone. I tell them I will not leave. They are not happy with me or my adamant demeanor. I am like a bulldog standing up for myself out of pure outrage. Outrage at my painful life and all the abuse I've encountered along the way. Finally the director of the program comes and says, "You raised so much hell I had to come out."

I see my life as a healing process, not as a mental illness. I lived in fear of becoming a bag lady for much of my life. I was so deeply saturated in hate and pain. I brought upon myself violence, shame, poverty and, for a while, homelessness as a teen. Then I began a very intentional spiritual path towards healing. This inner journey has been the core of my life and it continues to be my focus. It has been thwarted, diverted, and dismissed. It has been a long convoluted road. However, each step has taken me to the next. Each step is a puzzle piece.

I am sitting here at my desk in the nicest home I have ever provided for myself and my son. I marvel at the distance I have traveled to achieve the one major life goal I have ever had: the goal of sanity and choice. I am at a place I never thought I could get to, but always knew I was meant to go.

There were years when I had paralyzing depression where I just couldn't move. Now I take care of myself, I get up, I have a plan for the day. I exercise and meditate, and I make really good food to nourish my body. What I want you to know is that this is really the warrior's journey. Although it has been pain-filled and arduous, it has been most rewarding.

I remember denouncing God:
I was five years old
and I was being kicked by work boots while
I was on the kitchen floor.

Interviews by Cassandra Nudel, Cynthia Power & Ken Moore; Photographs by Cassandra Nudel

Joni, tell us about your childhood, the conditions that you recall.

This is the moment when I remember denouncing God: I was five years old and I was being kicked by work boots while I was on the kitchen floor. I seethed with hatred for my parents, my life and myself. I spent time each day fantasizing about harming — even killing — my parents. I did everything I can to make their lives equally miserable. At the age of 13, they put me in a mental hospital.

The people who ran the hospital were really sicker than the patients. I was tied to the mattress with leather restraints at my feet, waist and hands for two weeks at a time. I was left naked in a padded room for days. There was drugs and sex and lies and rape.

I was ordered to write my crimes one thousand times: "I will not walk around without a bra" and "I will not kiss a boy."

How do parents have the ability to incarcerate their children in psychiatric hospitals? Did your parents have to go through some kind of process to put you there?

All they had to do in those days was bring me there. I was a minor. I remember I was tripping on LSD and I had some friends over and we were being rowdy and my parents said, "We're going." I said, "Where are we going?" and they took me to the hospital.

My second hospitalization at age 15 lasted an entire year. There was electro-shock treatment against my will and it was probably the scariest thing I have ever lived through – and that includes living on the streets of Chicago.

I had one great accomplishment at the mental hospital. A friend of mine brought drugs in and the doctor found out. The doctor decided he would give me "the truth serum" sodium pentathol so I would rat out my friends. I prepared my mind and told myself what I wanted him to know: not the truth. I outmaneuvered the truth serum! That was a rewarding rebellion.

I was in the hospital for a year when I got out; the only reason I got out was because my aunt came to see me. She went back to my mother and said, "You need to get her out of there."

How did you continue on through that time?

I was completely full of rage. That was what kept me going and helped me get through it. I stayed out all night and ran away a number of times. I stayed high until I was 21. Sex and drugs and anything I could do to dull the pain.

I almost died a few times and wanted to die more often than not. I'm not a suicidal-depressed person. I'm a homicidal-depressed person. I mean, I'm not going to go kill somebody, but there's that tendency. There are the depressed people who sit in a corner and hate themselves; I hated everyone else.

Can you tell us the story of how you left Chicago?

So, I am 17 years old and I am working at a furniture store. One day this rugged mountain man walks in carrying a beautiful, handmade, stained-glass lamp. My mission is this: *Get the hell out of Chicago.* I am open to all opportunities. We talk and flirt. He is going back to Colorado and I make sure he wants me to go with him.

We have some interesting times. We live in a teepee in winter. We have a bridge on the property and carry water over it and chop wood. I do leatherwork and he makes stained glass. We have a white owl who lives there and he does his owl thing each night. We have an outside wood-burning cook stove and I bake bread on Sundays. It is awesome and beautiful and I love it for the time I have it.

When did you start moving toward self-awareness?

As an adult, I became a proficient gypsy, always moving when something finished badly – and that was often. I wound my way around the country, trying to find myself, to find some way to have it all be different. What I discovered was it could not be different unless I could accept life exactly how it was. I am a high-strung, opinionated, outgoing introvert. That's my nature. I can't change that. I spent years trying to not be that way only to discover I can't and I have to accept myself as I am. If I accept who I am as I am, only then can change happen.

What our culture calls "people with mental illness," others call shamans or visionaries – people who have easy access to these other realms. The first time I tried transcendental meditation, I had an out-of-body experience. When the teacher came into the room, I literally slammed back into my body from that other place. For the next six months, twice a day, I meditated with the busiest, most chattering, most judgmental mind possible. I learned that just sitting in meditation through that kind of mind-blaring chatter, results are being produced anyway. That was the beginning.

Each piece on my road to healing presented itself from here. I was in an Emotional Release class in massage school, and I volunteered to be worked on in front of the group. The instructor brought my anger to the surface through bodywork techniques. He did this with the intention of bringing to light and releasing the blinding affect of the male influences in my life. The hatred and unworthiness issues surfaced so deeply and unexpectedly that they scared me. My violent emotional release also affected the men in the class. But I must tell you, to have access to those inner demons with the skill of a trained professional guiding me into and through was the beginning of my liberation and healing.

When a place on your body is massaged, very specific events can come up to be released. I made a list of all my traumas, and I sat down and one by one I released them. Some took longer than others. I could literally feel the space and room that comes from releasing those pains. For the first time, I had hope that healing was possible.

I was mean for a long time. I was mad for a long time. I led my life from hatred, revenge and denial. My rage has served me well, but it has also caused me pain and suffering. Then I started watching my thinking and the energy from which I lived – rage-filled, blaming, resentful and entitled. Very slowly, over many years, as I was exposed to healing, I started taking responsibility for my thinking and vibrations.

I made a list of all my traumas,
and I sat down and one by one I released
them... I could literally feel the space and
room that comes from releasing those pains.

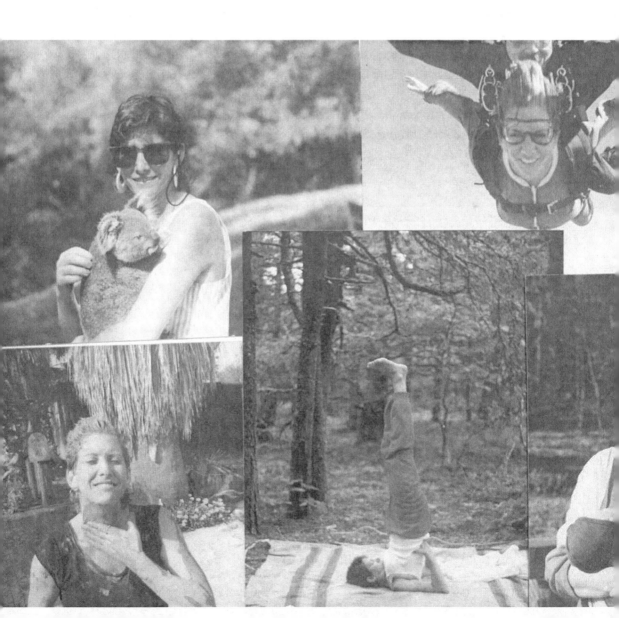

What do you mean when you talk about "vibrational wellness"?

We get what we give, but we don't get it from anyone else. We get it from the giving of it. What we give to others vibrationally, we also give to ourselves. If my vibration is resentful towards someone else, I am resentful towards myself. I realized that if I go out into the world pissing and moaning and blaming, then what I'm going to get is more opportunity to piss and moan and blame. I wrangle with my mind and sometimes I still have to remind myself: *Look at what I'm thinking. Look at who I'm being. Look at what I'm feeling. What vibrations am I putting out? Is this really what I want?* I began learning to shift these negative energies into something else – kindness to myself, behaving in loving ways to myself and doing kind, self-enriching things.

One thing led to the next through my intention to heal. I came to realize that I am responsible for everything in my universe. I learned to take responsibility for everything – even the stuff I had no control over and was a "victim" of. If a guy slams on his brakes in front of me and I have to slam on my brakes and I get angry at him, I feel that anger and I don't want to feel that. It became apparent that this was the only way to experience freedom, to be open to a life where I could make choices for myself instead of living the default life I was born into. If I change my thoughts, I will feel better whatever the external circumstances. This has been the hardest thing I've ever had to do.

Recovery can require time, hard work, and using some kind of a program. It seems as though some people think recovery is just going to happen.

I thought that for years, too. I was waiting for my life to change. What it takes to flourish is an attitude: *I'm not living this way. I don't care what it takes.* But it is not an attitude that you can just adopt. It must come from the core of one's being and a deep and unfailing commitment to personal evolution no matter what. We have to make conscious choices so we are not left as victims in our own lives. This is the warrior's choice. It is hard, painful and arduous, but the time will pass anyway so we may as well use it for our health and well being.

So many of us are given these medications that make us gain a lot of weight. You obviously have done a lot to get yourself in shape. How did you do that? How did you get yourself to exert the effort that was necessary?

I feel stable. I still swing up and down, but I know how to take care of myself.

There came a point when I just said, "I'm not taking anything that makes me gain weight. I'm not taking anything that gives me headaches. I'm not taking anything that has sexual side effects. I'm not doing it." I started being my own care provider. I started teaching my psychiatrists that they were my helpers. I was not just going to submit to what they thought was going to work for me. My doctor found a medication that worked for me. There are no side effects, so even though it is not perfect, I feel stable. I still swing up and down, but I know how to take care of myself.

Is there anything else about your journey you want us to know?

Yes, the story of my car. Years ago, I was going to visit my mother and I asked a friend of mine if I could leave my car in his driveway. Our agreement was I would leave the key, but unless he was bleeding to death he would not drive the car. He dropped me off at the bus and I heard this loud, booming voice screaming inside me say: *Do not leave your car with him!* but I ignored it.

When I got back, of course, he had driven the car in the snow and crashed into a wall and the insurance had lapsed. It was totaled. After that, I promised myself I would learn to navigate my intuition and learn how it spoke to me. I spent a year or so figuring out how my instincts worked and how the universe guided me.

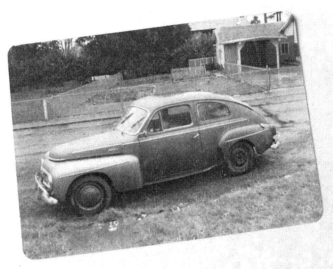

Intuition is always accurate. The challenge is deciphering what voices you are hearing. The mind is loud, obnoxious, and opinionated. It is a challenge to get beyond that to the small quiet information that intuition offers. Learning intuition can save a lot of grief and bad choices. I was mad at my friend for four years. Then I saw that he is the reason I embarked on my experiment to see how intuition speaks to me.

Let me tell you about how Nicolas, my son, came to be. A year before I met his father I had a dream about them both. We were in a park and I was getting ice cream for them. I knew they were my family and I knew the child's name was Nicolas. When I woke up, I thought I would meet someone who had a two-year-old child named Nicolas – because I knew I was never going to have children.

One day I was going to look at a place for rent. A man opened the door, and the first thought that went through my head was: *If I was ever going to have children, it would be with this man.* It turned out to be true. When I learned I was pregnant, I just freaked out because I had to decide: *Am I going to stay on psychiatric medication or am I going to have this child?* I was beside myself. I was hysterical. Then I realized who it was. It was Nicolas. I was meant to have him and I knew that.

Pregnancy did me good hormonally but after two years of breast feeding, I became terribly unstable, and wanted to go back on medication. So Nicolas and I did a breast feeding week long letting-go plan. It was poignant and beautiful the way he, my angelic two-year-old, supported me by letting go so I could attend to my mental health. It is sad how my mental health challenges have taken their toll on all of us but, most importantly, on him who I love so deeply.

What our culture calls
"people with mental illness,"
others call shamans or visionaries.

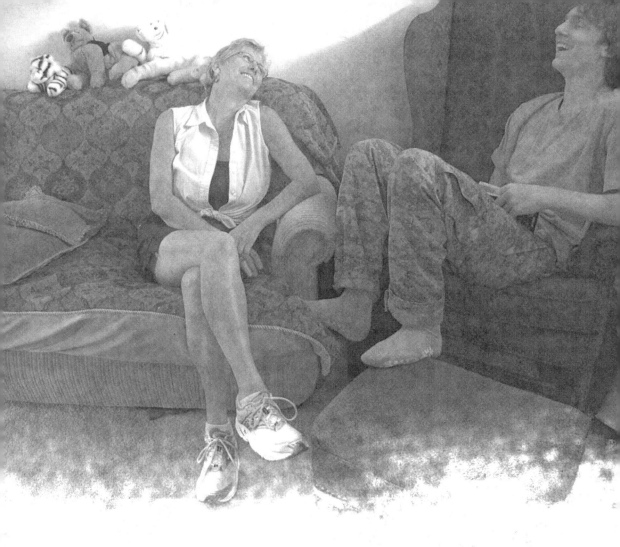

It sounds like you've had this amazing journey towards healing – going forward on faith and never knowing if you were going arrive somewhere better – and now in the past few years you've crossed a threshold and something is different.

I moved to Virginia seven years ago when my son was 11. I was intuitively guided with the help of an astrologer. She said anywhere within 100 miles of Woodbridge, Virginia, is energetically good for us.

I had $1,800 when we got on a Greyhound bus. We came to Charlottesville and we spent two weeks at the Salvation Army shelter. Even staying at the Salvation Army was better than where we'd been. It was so liberating.

Since moving here, I broke a record twice: We lived in one dwelling for three years and then we lived in a townhouse for four years. This is my home. I love it here. I can relax into my life.

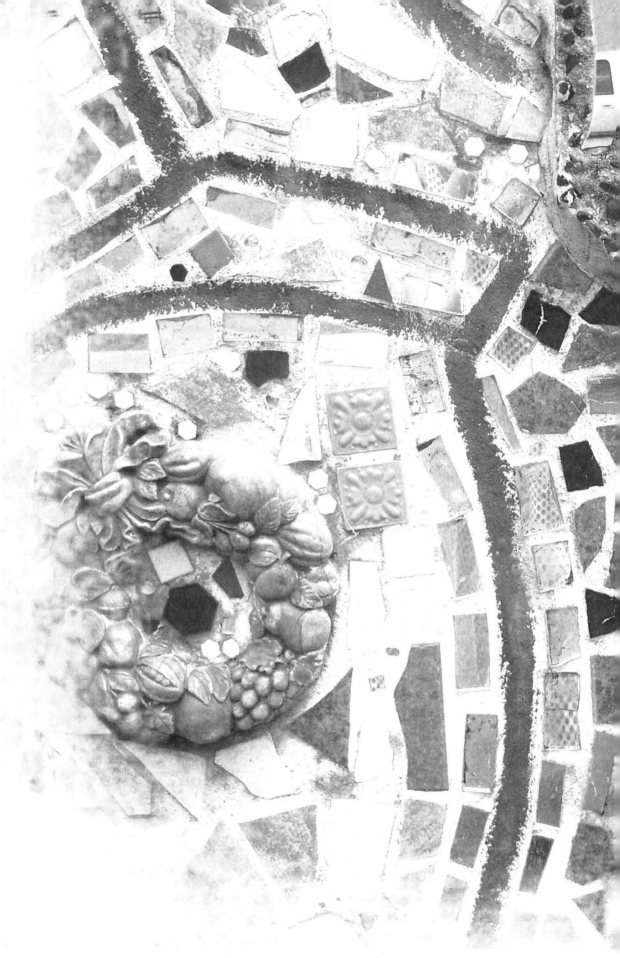

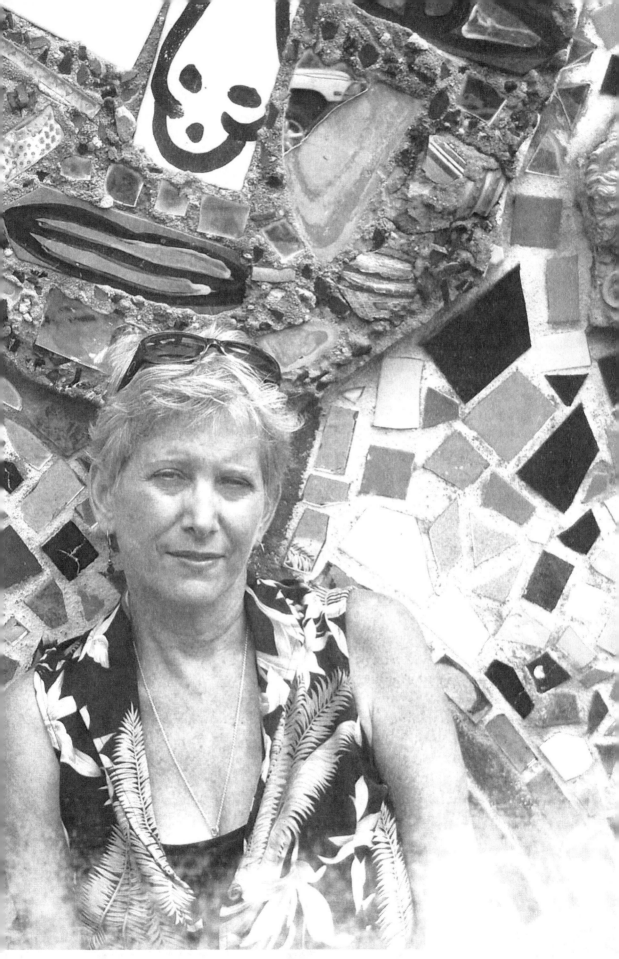

Intuition is always accurate.
The challenge is deciphering what voices
you are hearing.

I found my spiritual teacher Master Charles at a healing center nearby called Synchronicity. As soon as I got there, I was enthralled. I knew I was home. Master Charles created and teaches high tech-meditation. It's out-of-the-box healing through brain balancing frequencies. We use headphones and listen to technology created to literally balance the brain. When I began, I would sit down to meditate and the sounds and music were so powerful, I could feel my cells responding. If I am late in the day to meditate, my body calls me; I feel like I am being sucked back into a tunnel. My cells are calling me, needing their nourishment.

I am who I am today because my brain is being balanced with this technology. I have been at my job a year and three quarters — a lifetime record for me.

Do you communicate with your parents now?

I never in a million years thought I could, but there came a time when I wanted to have my dad in my life. It was clear that I was going to have to take responsibility for my actions regardless of what he did or didn't do. I sent him a letter and I apologized for all the malicious things I had ever done to him. That created a bridge. Now we talk regularly, and he opened up a college fund for Nicolas. I am grateful for our relationship. My mom and I started working on our relationship in 1982. It took us some years to purge all the guilt and manipulations we used. We worked hard and diligently and it paid off. We talk regularly now and we both feel love, appreciation, and gratitude for our relationship.

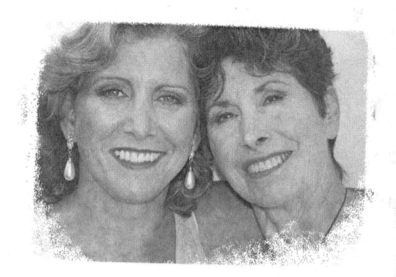

When you were growing up, did you know all along that the problem wasn't you – it was the circumstances around you?

I *did* know that, and I was really mad about it and nobody would hear me. When I was in sixth grade, I was forced to see the school psychologist because I was uncooperative and angry. They said it was my problem – not looking at the fact that my parents were beating me and telling me how worthless I was. I was diagnosed with bipolar disorder at 14, but I didn't believe them. The "professionals" saw themselves as saviors doing the best they could with such a troubled child. It never dawned on them that the physical and emotional abuse might have triggered the symptoms causing the diagnosis.

I use the words "chemical imbalance." Chemical imbalance is a condition I have; it is not the dominant force in my life. It is statistically proven that when a child is abused for more than a six month period, their chemistry changes.

I see my life as a healing process, not as a mental illness. There are still days when I feel hopeless, depressed, and apathetic. I have not eliminated the chemistry or my humanity. The gamut of emotions is a human experience. I do not think of myself as someone with an illness, but I must address the imbalance. I maintain my self-care, psychiatry, exercise, proper nutrition, and connectedness with others. I can swing from the rafters sometimes. When this happens, I remember all I know about people and life from a spiritual perspective. What goes up must come down.

I SEE THAT ALL THIS TIME,

through everything I was doing, my sense of self was developing,

like laying a stone path, one stone at a time.

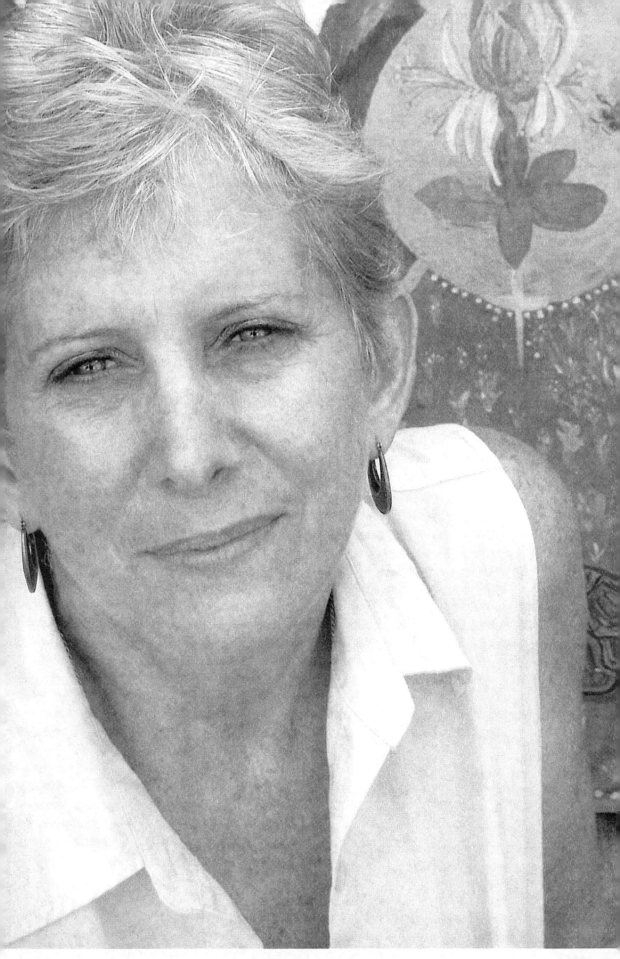

TRACY'S STORY

My fire has been spiritual.

At 16, I first became spiritually frozen.
After someone told me that there was such a thing as
"UNPARDONABLE SIN,"
I was traumatized and sick for a long time.

I felt frozen in time.

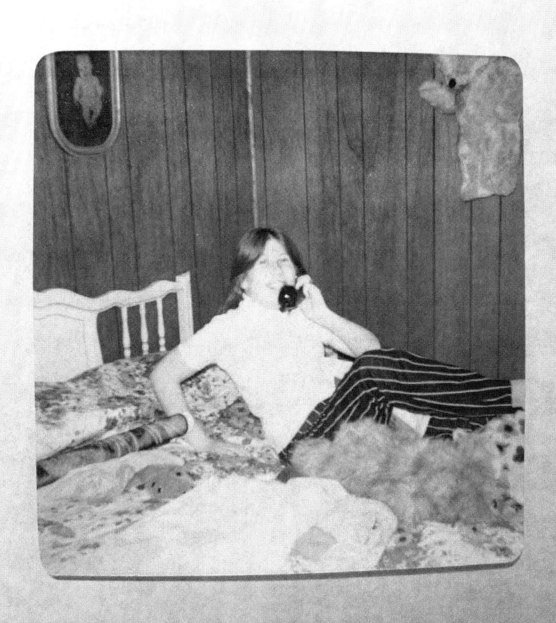

I was

fighting some kind of spiritual battle. That's how it started. I went to places in my mind that were frightening. I lost so much of my life during that time period.

Religious issues were the first trigger in my life. I was looking out at the living world from within my very small space. Now when I look at the stars, the mountains, the sky, I know there is so much more. This great thing that caused all the many universes, this world, and other worlds is so much bigger and so much better than the boxes we have created here, in this one tiny little place, on this one little planet.

I believe in the mystery of it all. I believe we are connected to every other thing from the dirt of the ground, to the sands of the sea, to the gravity that takes hold of us all. If I said that God is all about what goes on in a building, I would be lying. We are all more alike than we are different, and everywhere I go, and anywhere I've ever been, I have seen this to be true, time and time again.

I've come to realize that there was never anything to be forgiven for. There is only a continuum of mystery and sorrow followed by joy. I can see that there is no end. There was a beginning for me even before my birth here, but there is no end to the questions, the wonder, and the wandering in the wilderness at times. I believe we see through a glass darkly now, and in some awesome way that I can't explain, I find comfort in this. I find hope.

I grew up in a very wholesome coal mining camp where we were very sheltered from the world. If I had never encountered mental health struggles, I might have lived a life that was quite insulated. I might not have broadened my mind. Sometimes we have to go through our own personal hell to come to a place of reckoning. Though I walked through horrible and scary places, I have found a peace in knowing what kindles my spirit. Some of the frozen times did not offer very beautiful views, though some of them did.

I would ask, "Do you think I'm going to lose my mind totally?"

And she would reply, "I don't know."

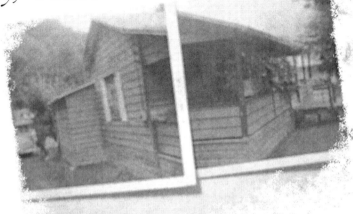

Interviews by Bev Ball & Debra Knighton; Photographs by Cassandra Nudel & Brian Parrish

Tracy, how does your story begin?

In the coalfields where I was raised, people worked hard. My grandfather who raised me was wise beyond his formal sixth-grade education. He went to work in the mines at age 12. He loved me deeply, though he didn't verbally express this to me very often. As I went on my way during my pre-teen years, he made some predictions about my life: I would learn the hard way. He was so right.

It was the summer of 1979 when I moved in with my aunt, uncle, and two cousins in Virginia. I took a job at the local newspaper office. I corrected the copy for the paper manually – as computers were not used for such work in those days. I loved the job; I netted about $100 a week. One day while working on the paper, I began to have disturbing thoughts. They were spiritual in nature. Each day, the thoughts came more and more frequently, and eventually, I was unable to pay attention to my work. My mother took me to the local hospital. This visit marked the first of several emergency room visits that were to come later in my life.

In the fall of 1981, a pastor friend drove me to Huntington, West Virginia, where I began my college career at Marshall University. My mind was opened to possibilities and dreams in those days. I remained well throughout the years I spent on Marshall's campus. I held work-study jobs and made several friends who are dear friends to this day. I felt I was in control of my life for once. I actually believed I was happy for a time.

But some years later when I ended up in Charleston, staying with my old college friend in her very small trailer home, I was a total mess. I was so sick that I wasn't able to do much of anything but wander. My friend was stunned and afraid for me. She had never seen me that way throughout our years at college. She would say, "I don't know what to do. I don't know what's going to happen to you." I would ask, "Do you think I'm going to lose my mind totally?" And she would reply, "I don't know." My mother and cousin came to get me and we traveled to Cleveland, Ohio. I went into the hospital almost immediately. It was a fine facility. A fine psychiatric ward. I was given a diagnosis of severe agitated depression.

I will simply tell you that in those days I was doing lots of running. I was lonely and lost. I traveled to Cambridge, Ohio, where I was hired to work as a speech therapist in a private school for handicapped children. My dog was my only companion in the empty apartment where I lived. I thought I was going to settle in and fill my big apartment with furniture and live happily ever after, but I began to think a lot. And write a lot. As I wrote, I lost sleep. I began writing during working hours. One day, I was simply asked to sign some papers, gather my things, and leave.

Time passed. No job. No money. No furniture. No home. Back to the fine hospital I went. More therapy. More classes. Eventually the doctors diagnosed me as manic-depressive, and I was released.

My cousin used to come and drag me out of bed, make me get into the shower, and take me out to lunch. I really don't know what I would have done in those days had it not been for my mother and my cousin who encouraged me and showed such compassion for my situation. Every single day I forced myself out of bed though I was so afraid to even face the light of day. I would shower and dress, then walk a few blocks downtown to a cathedral, and help prepare food to feed the hungry by midday.

I was so afraid. Still every single day, I continued to feel the fear, but move forward. As I look back on that time period, I've come to realize that the initiative I took by forcing myself out of bed every morning, bathing, and then walking downtown to the cathedral, marked a turning point in my life. I was driven, even if by my own fears.

When did things change?

One day in the summer of 1990, my mom and I got a phone call that my grandmother had been in a car accident. We went to the hospital and stood by her bed. I remember kneeling down next to her ear and saying, "Nanny, it's OK. You have to go now. Thank you for all that you have done for my life. I love you so." And with that, my grandmother died at 3pm that summer day.

After my grandmother's funeral, I made the decision that even if my friends all knew I had been hospitalized, and even if I never had managed my life well to that point, I had to start over. Some way or another, I had to start again and make a life for myself.

I traveled back to our empty homestead in the coalfields of West Virginia. I went off all of my medications and flushed them down the toilet. The doctor had been prescribing lithium to me and upping the dosages every time I visited, until I became toxic. The doctor didn't know me. I saw her for 30 minutes at a time. I'd tell her a little bit about my life, and she would up the lithium. That was it. I got angry and decided, "No more!" When I came home to West Virginia I felt pretty good, very creative and happy and alive.

Out of the blue, an old high school girlfriend called to tell me she heard that I was back home and she had in mind a man she wanted me to meet. I told her that I had absolutely no interest in meeting anyone at that time—I was preparing to go back to school in the spring, and I wanted to concentrate on nothing more.

When I met Sam, he was like a step back in time for me. That day I felt just exactly the way I wanted to feel. I was with an old friend from high school and I had just met a really good-looking, sweet guy who reminded me of home folks. He was very down-home. I was enamored by his musical talent and his sweetness. It was kind of a love at first sight thing for me. I said, "This is it. This guy is it."

When I was really sick, I always used to say, "I want to be my old self again." I didn't realize there was a new self that I could become.

Time passed.
No job. No money. No furniture. No home.
Back to the fine hospital I went.

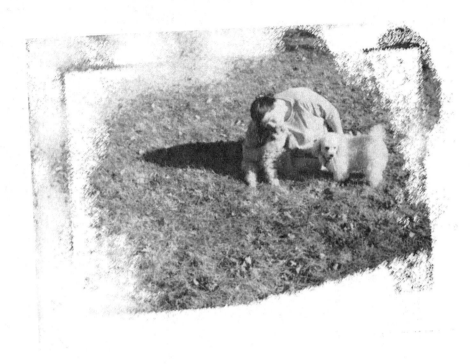

And you decided to get married?

In July of '93 I began to make all sorts of arrangements for a church wedding. I was to have friends from back home in the coalfields as bridesmaids and singers, and my best friend from college was to be my maid of honor. I was flying high. I simply busied myself with much to do and then… Wham! I fell apart from the stress of it all. I began to feel trapped. I began to fear being married. I ended up in the hospital.

But he was still there for you throughout this whole thing?

He cried and he begged me to come home to him. The time passed and I felt better. I came home to my fiancé, and I went to see a wonderful psychiatrist in a lovely town in Virginia. He remains my doctor to this day.

My dear cousin and my mother decided to plan a small family wedding for us in a lovely park nearby. It was not fancy. No bridesmaids. My cousin's friend provided us with pale pink roses. I always wanted a red velvet cake and my little cousin got up early that morning and made a red velvet cake from scratch. It was the driest cake in the world but it was beautiful, *beautiful*. Sam and I had our little wedding on October 16 of 1993. My cousin was killed in a car accident six months later.

My husband is very much the same yesterday, today, and tomorrow. He's the same kind of guy all the time, and he helps keep my feet on the ground. I haven't been in the hospital since 1993 when I got married.

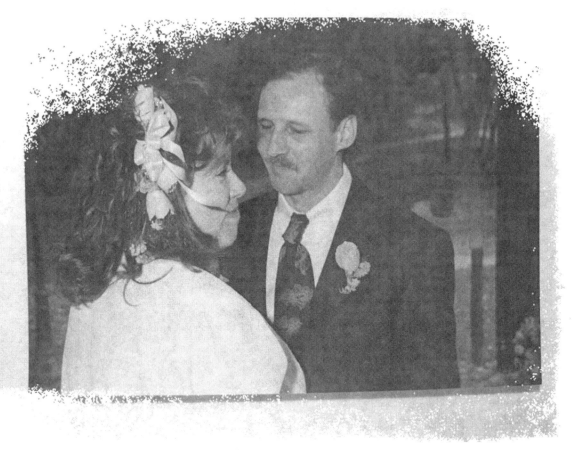

What was your experience with foster children?

I always knew I wanted to foster children the way my grandparents had fostered me. I wanted to offer some child a softer place to fall. My husband and I were foster parents from 1999 to 2004. I loved each and every child that came through our door. We adopted one daughter in heart, and she stayed with us past the age of 18. In September of 2006, our gal took off into the world again to make a life for herself. We love her so and continue to be available for her and her sister always.

I feel a great deal of guilt when I think back on some of the episodes I've experienced and what my family went through. I am learning to forgive myself. My foster daughter always knew that underneath it all I loved her more than life. I think that is was what held her to me. She knew that I would come out of it OK.

No matter what happened she would say, "This is *nothing* like the way it used to be before I came to you." My husband and I would get into an argument and she would say, "You guys are *funny*. You fight and make up so quickly; I don't pay any attention. I've seen much worse." I've come to believe that the good I did for her outweighs any grief she may have suffered because of the issues that tormented me from time to time. At least I believe it for this moment.

My husband is the same kind of guy all the time, and he helps keep my feet on the ground. I haven't been in the hospital since 1993 when I got married.

Looking back, how did your family react when you were first diagnosed?

When I was a kid, I didn't know I had a mental illness; I didn't even dream of such a thing. I didn't know what was going on. I would say to the doctors, "I have racing thoughts, and when I look down at my hands, I don't feel like they are mine anymore. I *know* they are my hands, but they don't look like my hands." The doctors would write on my charts that I was delusional.

My grandparents were just terribly afraid for me and didn't know what to do, but they stuck by me through everything. When I was a child, my grandpapa didn't attend church, but he taught me the psalms and old hymns. My grandmother was a rock for me. Through the years we spent many days chatting about life and love. She taught me grace.

My mom was there through the most difficult times of my mental illness. She always told me, "You're going to be well someday; it's going to be OK." Even though we didn't live together, we remained in constant contact. My father was not as supportive. His attitude was, "You look OK, so you ought to be OK. You've just got to use will power." My father told me to join the rest of the human race and get a job.

My family stayed afraid during the worst of my illness. Sometimes they were sharp with me because of fear. I think my family sometimes had *empathy* and *sympathy* confused. They thought they were being empathetic, when really it was more like pity. Now, I try to teach them. I tell them how I'm feeling, and I tell them, "Don't pity me."

What is the work you're doing to resurrect the Turning Point program?

I never knew Turning Point existed. I had been working as a desk clerk at a local hotel, but I had problems with arthritis in my knees. One day I was taking my dogs home from the vet and one of my dearest friends in town came out and said "Oh, *you* are the person! You have to do this job." She told me, "They

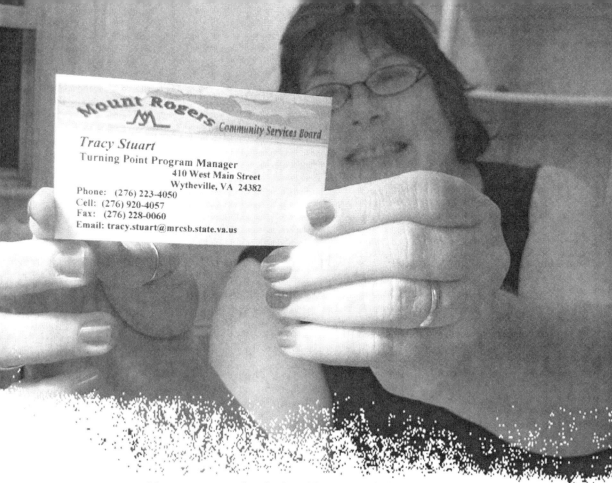

want to hire someone who deals with a mental illness and can become a peer support person. The only thing is you have to be willing to share your story with people."

In December of 2007, I was hired as the manager of Turning Point, a program within our local mental health system. The first thing I did was train to become a Peer Support Specialist and learn all about mental health wellness and recovery. Peer Support Specialists are a whole new approach in the mental health system. We are people who have managed our own mental health issues; we have been through the darkness and learned how to cope. Now we work with others who are going through similar things. Our life experience gives us what is needed to do this job. Now we're starting support groups, we're teaching recovery, and we have an acute care center. I am going to be a point person for the other Peer Support Specialists. I don't know how this happened, but I got nominated to be vice-chair of a mental health recovery committee, so now I'm the vice-chair.

Turning Point is a perfect name for our program because we all come to a turning point in our lives, a crossroads where we have to decide which way to go. I've got a mountain to climb here in southwest Virginia, but I hope there are some people who will climb that mountain with me.

Thank you, Tracy, for what you're doing to revive the mental health recovery movement in southwest Virginia. What is the big message you would like to get out there?

My goal in my job now is to tell other people that there is hope. I tell my staff, "We are salespeople of hope." I do believe in faith and love, but if you don't have hope, you don't get out of bed in the morning.

I know there is hope for people, because in my darkest hours, I wasn't getting out of bed, I wasn't showering, I was closing off the light to my room, closing the windows and shutting the blinds, and I didn't think I was ever going to be released. When you're going through it, you think it's never going to end. I told God, "If you get me out of here, I'm never going to come to this place again."

And I never have.

In your darkest hours, back then or now, what's helped you to carry on?

I didn't always *feel* hope, but I think that any time I get out of bed in the morning and put one foot in front of the other, that is expressing hope. Usually if I get up and push myself on days when I don't feel well, I find that there's something I can accomplish that day that allows me to go to bed feeling better about myself. It's hope that gives us faith. It's hope that gets us going. So I just kind of wait to see what's around the corner.

I believe actual recovery has to come from within. You have to do the work; you have to do it. When I was first hospitalized, I was afraid and I would say, "Do you think I'm going to be OK?" The staff would assure me that I would be. But then there came a day when I would say "Do you think I'll be OK?" and they would say, "What do you think?" I had to learn for myself that I was going to get through this. I had to decide for myself that someday, today, I could be OK.

There was a time when I wouldn't look anybody in the eye. I always had to look down. Now I've learned how to be myself and relax a little more. I was obsessively concerned with getting things done. Now my vision for middle age is to just enjoy life. I want to have more joy in the next years of my life than I ever did before. It's OK to not finish a project.

Twenty years ago when I was so vulnerable to people, I worried about things that I don't think about today. I would become so stressed about what to wear to my doctor's office that I didn't know if I could even manage to go. There's something about aging that's a blessing.

Was there an "aha" moment in any part of your journey?
A moment of enlightenment?

Anyone who's dealt with a mental illness has really walked through fire. We deal with things at a deeper level. The struggles are spiritual. It's more than just: "How do I get my bills paid today?"

When I was younger, I really believed I had committed some unpardonable sin, and I was frozen in that belief for a long time. I go so far as to think that it is abusive and neglectful to fill a youngster's mind with such fear, to fill *anyone's* mind with such fear, to use fear as a means to try to "save a lost soul."

Many years later, when I took foster children into my home, some children arrived whose parents were pastors. They came from a denomination that taught the way to "save souls" was to scare people into the "kingdom." I had been through all my fear and obsession many years ago, and now I had the opportunity to share love with these beautiful children who were downtrodden by a group that thought they had the secret to all of God's glory.

In college I had a mentor who was my very best friend. She was also somewhat manic-depressive – with an IQ that was out of this world. During all those many tough years when I was sick with the misery of guilt and worry that I had done something unforgivable, she used to tell me that she goes through questioning her faith cyclically. She would say to me, "In the end, after all your questioning and wondering, it all comes down to one thing. You either believe or you don't believe in something more than what is here in front of you." And I really do believe. That's what it all comes down to.

My "aha moments" have come in cycles. I believe that pieces of our lives fit together like a puzzle in ways that we don't often see until many years later. I believe in the mystery. I just have no way of explaining it to a non-believer,

The thing I've learned through mental illness is this: I've learned how to grow up. I've had to grow into myself. In that sense, I am transformed.

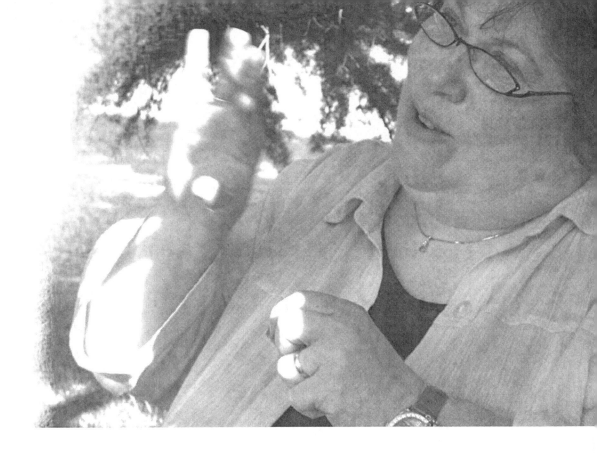

other than to tell my own personal story, which is that my prayers have been answered. In one way or another things kind of tie in together and I look back later and say, *Now I know why that happened!*

In what ways has your experience with mental illness permanently changed you—for better or for worse?

The thing I've learned through mental illness is this: I've learned how to grow up. I've had to grow into myself. In that sense, I am transformed.

My mental illnesses have enlightened me, so to speak. My faith is stronger. God is in all of us and we are all bits and pieces of God, just like the sand and the ocean. We are all tiny grains of sand, but we are all integral pieces of the universe.

There is a quote from C.S. Lewis: "We cannot possibly have joy without sorrow."

I believe actual recovery has to come from within.

When I was first hospitalized, I was afraid
and I would say, *"Do you think I'm going to be OK?"*
But then there came a day when I would say
"Do you think I'll be OK?"

and they would say,
"What do you think?"

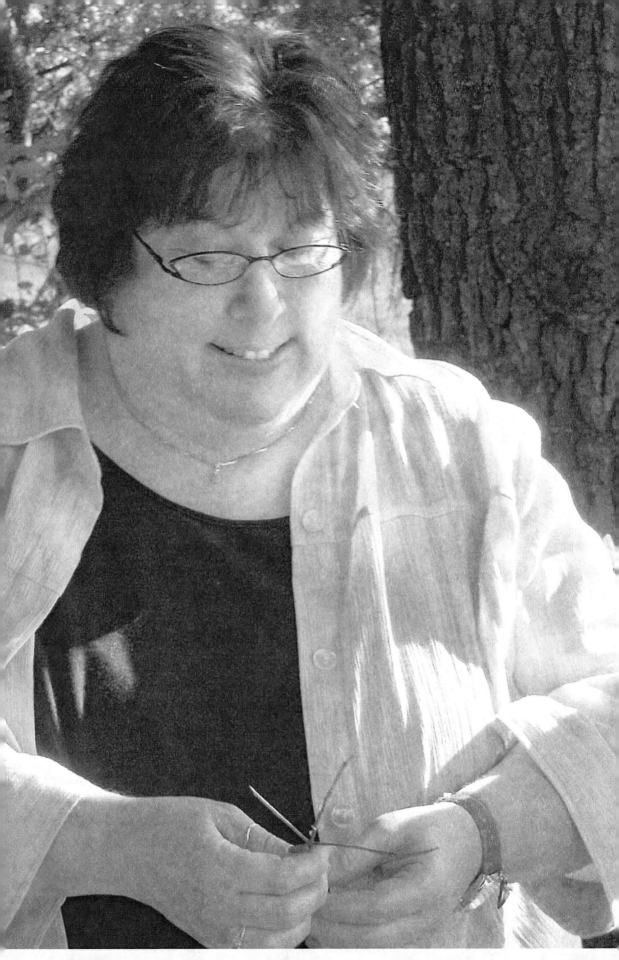

Burning Questions

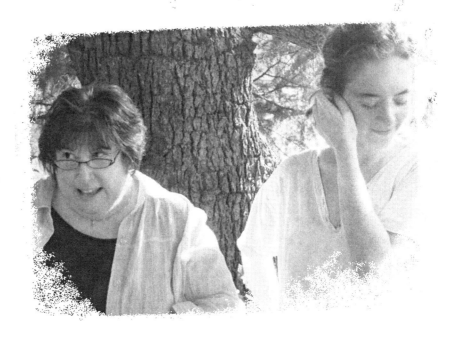

What's in your wellness toolbox?

Debra: I wish I had learned earlier that there were things that I could do to help myself. I have some control over whether I get better or not. I am amazed at how food and exercise can affect my thinking and my emotions. If I'm not out walking and I'm eating sugar, somehow things just start to fall apart. Hugging my kids and my husband helps more than you would think. It takes me to a different place where I feel like there is meaning in life. God blessed me with two very affectionate boys and a very affectionate husband. Medication is another key tool for me. Some people don't need it, but I've tried to go off medication, and I've found that it is not a good idea for me.

Sometimes I don't feel like doing the things that help me, and I cycle down until I realize that I just have to do them in order to get back on track. That's something I think I learned a little bit late.

Tracy: I like to touch things. If I'm really stressed, I like to have something in my hand. I like to dig in the dirt or play in the mud; I love the feel of the cool ground. Planting flowers or bushes helps me to come alive from within. I also like to sit in the back row of the dark theater, and nobody knows where I am. It's really good to have a place to go to get away from everything. There were times when I felt like the walls were closing in on me, and I took myself to a hotel and checked into a comfortable room for the night. In extremely stressful situations, that is something I've done to quiet my mind and spirit.

I don't think anyone can tell you what to do to feel better. It has to be whatever works for you.

Carla: I wrote throughout my psychosis. I felt tremendous pressure in my head and writing helped relieve that pressure. Another thing that helped me get through the dark time was physical activity. When I was going in and out of reality, I would just shovel mulch into my flower borders. My wellness tools are exercising, using stress reduction techniques, having some down time to myself every day, eating a well balanced diet, drinking water, and journaling. When I was extremely busy and quit taking the time to use my wellness tools, my mental health symptoms returned.

Joni: There is a tool I use to release negative emotions and allow them to leave the body. It can be found at **releasetechnique.com**. I made a list of the traumatic events in my life. Then I went through the entire list over a period of nine months and have diminished the emotion so it does not reside in my body or cells. Cellular memory is often taking up space and not allowing for new and different experiences of life. When this stockpile of unwanted emotion is reduced, there is actually room for more flow through our lives.

Myra: I changed my relationship with mental health providers. I began to look at people who were providing treatment for me as co-partners instead of people trying to tell me what to do. I took their advice into consideration and then made my own choice about what's best for me. I began to direct my own treatment.

Lauren: I find a private and safe place with another trusted person, and we take turns expressing our thoughts and feelings. This supports me to figure out the root of the distress and how to grow beyond it. The other thing I do is go for a walk or do something fun which takes my attention off distress and onto the present moment. If I am in the present, I am well.

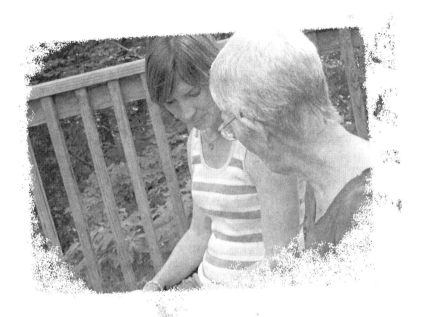

What do you wish someone had told you when you were first diagnosed? What would you want to tell someone else?

Tracy: Don't just go home and take a pill and think that the best you can do is to work at McDonald's. I *know* there are people who deal with mental health issues who are brilliant people. They are working wonderful jobs, and having families, and living what most would envision as a normal life.

Pat Deegan is one of my idols. She is one of the people who was told to go home and take a pill, and maybe she'd work at McDonald's someday. Now she has a PhD. She is one of my favorite speakers and a pioneer in the mental health recovery movement. In her writing she says: You can only do something for so long before your body is going to want to do something else. If you sit in a corner and stare at a wall long enough, eventually you're going to get tired of that. This comes from a spiritual drive; it comes from within. Our healing is within us.

When I was terribly sick and non-functioning, I needed to know there was hope to replace my fears. Know that there is hope no matter what. If you grasp this concept early on, you can walk through the fires and the dark places of the soul and come out washed and untouched by burns.

Debra: This is the most important thing for me: What's in my life today isn't necessarily what's going to be in my life tomorrow. Things can change overnight or things can change in a week. When I'm in the midst of depression and feeling like I really need to cut or I don't want to live anymore, I've gotten better at saying, *Depression never lasts forever; it may last a few months, but it doesn't last forever.* I've gotten better at knowing that life is ever-changing and that God will bring people into my life who will change how I look at things.

Things are going to change and in ways I could never expect. That is a fact. Things change for people who think they've got it all together and things change for people who think their world has fallen apart completely. When I was first getting out of the hospital and I was totally afraid of the world, I never could have imagined that someday I was going to have a job I love that is totally suited for me. The message I want to give people is to sit through the pain. It's uncomfortable, but it's guaranteed that life is going to change.

Michelle: I was told that my mental illness was degenerative; I would get worse with time and with age, and medication would help me to stay stable if my family took care of me. It's a pretty hopeless diagnosis from a doctor! If that's all people are being told, do you wonder why there so many suicides? Who wants to live like that? I wish that when I was first diagnosed the doctor had said, "There is life beyond your mental illness. You can still do all the things you want to do. It's just going to be a challenge."

You must have hope that there is life beyond that front door; there is life beyond that TV set; there is life beyond the couch. You can go outside, even if it's just going for a walk. That's a start into recovery. You can set small goals for yourself and work towards those little goals, then begin to set bigger and bigger goals, and keep on working towards those goals.

I hope that doctors who read this book will learn to give us choices. Let us choose whether we want to sit on the couch or whether we want to go outside our front door. Don't force us onto the couch.

Joni: This is the good news and the bad news: Our wellness is our personal responsibility. Everything out there – all the support, caregivers, services, books and information – none of it can help if we are not in touch with ourselves and making choices from our truth. We have to ask the right questions, even when it comes to meds. Drive your psychiatrist mad with needing to know. *What does it do? How does it work? What results will it produce? What are the side effects?* Believe me, I've had many a therapist and psychiatrist that were not happy with me and all these questions. I've even had to fire a few. I've required partnership in my wellness.

Carla: Find something that helps you to get through the hard times. When I started to feel surreal and disconnected, I would do something physical. I would shovel mulch or work outside, and that would help me feel connected again.

One thing that's important to me is suicide prevention. I want for people to realize that there is hope. Your life is precious and you don't know what could have become of your life if you end it. It reminds me of the loss my family and the world suffered when my brother ended his life. Don't give up. Have hope. You will get through it.

Lauren: I would tell someone: your dreams can come true. There is great hope and expectation that you will recover and have a full life in the community. I expect nothing less of you. Keep your dreams in focus and direct your energy and intelligence to accomplishing them.

Crisis is an opportunity for growth, even in the midst of overwhelming circumstances. There are many people who have used their time with mental health struggles to explore new options and gain new understandings. You can learn to manage your vulnerabilities and become less susceptible to the pressures that cause the severe emotional distress.

Myra: I wish someone would have given me a glimmer of hope. As much medicine as was prescribed to me, I wish someone had prescribed just a little bit of hope. They didn't tell me much; only that I had a mental illness and that I was going to take medication for the rest of my life. It was very detrimental to me because I had a lot of dreams: I wanted to finish school, I wanted to go to college, I wanted to do many things in my life.

This is what I would say to other people along the journey:

> **You're an expert on yourself.** The doctors may be experts at medicine, but you've been living in your body for all these years and you are the expert on yourself. When my doctor tells me he wants me to take a medication, I talk to the pharmacist about it, I go on the Internet, I look up the information myself and then I come back and I say, "I know you want me to take this medicine; these are some concerns I have about what I've read. What do you say about this?"

> **You're a work-in-progress.** You don't just arrive overnight at the spot where you want to be. Living with a diagnosis is a process.

You have to constantly work on your recovery. You have to look at things like, "Did I get enough sleep last night?" or "Should I drink this much caffeine?" or other things that may affect your mental health.

Setbacks are a part of the recovery process. You're going to have setbacks along the way and that doesn't mean that you can't recover. It's important to learn all you can from the setbacks and move on.

There is a trap. There are times when you feel so good, you may think you don't need to go back and do the things that keep you well. For example, you may feel you don't need to take medicine anymore, or you don't need to see the doctor, or go to the support group. To me, this is a trap. T-R-A-P, trap! You're falling into a trap. Pay attention to what you're doing to stay well and keep doing those things.

Reach out to family and friends. I remember one time when I came out of the hospital and I wasn't doing very well, my aunt said, "Let me wash your hair for you." So she washed and dried and curled my hair. My cousin painted my toenails. That's something very simple that lifted me up. It didn't solve all my problems, but it made me feel that I was valued and in their own way they were saying, "You have our support."

Integrate into the community as much as possible. I don't really support housing where everyone who has a disability or a mental illness lives in one area. People need to know that you're their next door neighbor and you're part of the community. You may have a diagnosis, but you're just like them. You take your garbage to the same trash can they do. You water your yard just like they do.

Do not give up! Almost every job I had, I lost because of mental health problems, but I stayed in the game. All the heartache I went through was bringing me to the point where I am now. I tell people: Don't give up no matter what.

Hold onto hope and if you don't have hope, find someone who can hold it for you until you can hold it for yourself.

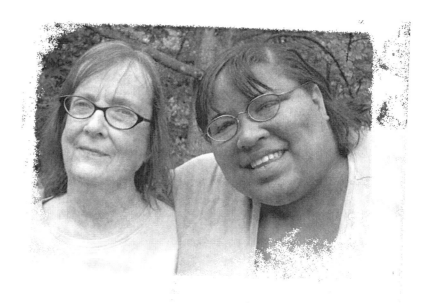

If you could change one thing about the mental health system...

Myra: Oh God, where do I start! One thing? All right, I'll start with one...

If you're having a physical crisis, they'll call an ambulance for you. If you're having a mental health crisis, police show up at your door ready to put you in handcuffs and haul you away. There's something wrong with that picture. The majority of people diagnosed with mental illness are not violent. The system is treating us like we're criminals – like there's something very criminal about having a mental illness.

Another thing I would change is what you hear when you first enter the mental health system: *This is wrong with you; this is wrong with you; this is wrong with you. You can't do this; you can't do this; you can't do this. Well, what the hell can I do? Is there anything right with me? Everything is wrong with me?* I would like the system to focus more on what's right with us – a more strengths-based approach.

I don't think that judges forcing people to have treatment is a good idea. Every time I've been forced to do something in my life, I haven't done the best job I could do, simply because I didn't want to do it. Mandatory outpatient commitment may look like it's getting results, but in the long term people aren't going to follow through.

Every year, they're coming up with a new way to restrain people. Instead of addressing the core of the problem, they invent a new chair to put people in restraints. There is no reason why all these people in psych wards have to be put on beds and have their hands and ankles strapped down and their movement restricted. My final thought is that the system needs to move to a model of "zero restraints." It's not radical thinking; it's been done in some other states.

Michelle: I wish there was some way to help caseworkers see that they're on the same level as we are. I should never be co-dependent on my caseworker. I should never feel, *Oh, I'm a hopeless case and I need you.* I wish there was a way for old-school caseworkers to be re-educated.

The housing office is telling me they want me to work. Medicaid is saying, "Well, if you go to work, we're not going to give you insurance, and by the way nobody else is going to give you insurance either!" *Hello!* No medication equals hospitalization!

It's a vicious cycle. It makes no sense, and it's ridiculous, but that's the way the system is built. If you want to cut the apron strings and go off Medicaid, there is no health insurance out there that can help. But you need health insurance to get your medication, or where are you going to be? The psychiatric hospital. So you have to stay on the apron strings and be taken care of by Medicaid, and if Medicaid says you can't work, too bad!

We need to get Medicaid, social services, housing offices, and mental health services to sit down and talk together and come up with one plan, one system, one program that works. That way we can become independent, work a job, make our own income, have a strong support system, and not get trapped in a revolving door going in and out of the hospital. The taxpayers are complaining that they're throwing away money by paying for us to go in and out of the hospital 9, 10, 12, 100 times.

We're like guinea pigs on a wheel, and we're constantly running. Well, I don't want to be on that wheel. I want to get off but they won't let me off. I wish the system would change.

Lauren: We need to understand that there is always a person inside even the most severely distressed individual. That person is usually frightened and may appear trapped in a different reality or temporarily lost in inner monologue. But that person understands more about what is going on than we realize. That person can often be reached by someone patient and skilled at engaging in dialogue. Peers who have been through similar experiences can help people traditional services can't reach. We need more human connection in the mental health system. We need to engage people in dialogue so they're not like I was: stuck in monologue.

When I was in the mental institution at 16, locked up and drugged up, I didn't trust authority figures. There was a psych tech who reached out to me, talking to me, every shift, five days a week, for three months. The night I was in the seclusion room, he volunteered to work all night and checked on me every 10 minutes. He was reaching for connection even though I was not able to return the attention. In the ensuing years, I came to realize the profound impact he'd had on me. I had never previously felt like I mattered — he taught me that I did.

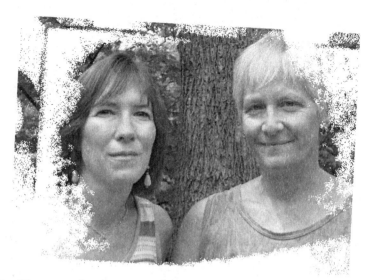

Can "mental illness" be learned?

Lauren: Whew! We've done a lot of interviews this weekend for *Firewalkers,* and I don't want to diminish what anyone else may have said, but I hear the term "mental illness" being spoken a lot. I don't call what I went through a *mental illness* or a *nervous breakdown.* I call it a *spiritual breakthrough.* I've spent a good 15 years in a long, slow process of learning that there was nothing wrong with me.

I hope the *Firewalkers* book turns the system inside out. I hope we can give people a glimpse of what it looks like to have a community where we're not judged by our diagnosis.

How do you get people to think differently? What if mental illness didn't exist? Can this thing called "mental illness" be learned? I know professionals who believe that it can, but they won't come out publicly and say it because it's a career buster. There's so much fear about saying something that radical. I get a little nervous saying it even in this group.

Carla: Sorry to interrupt. . . but what do you mean "mental illness can be learned"?

Lauren: Oppression comes from the outside and we internalize it. For example, growing up, my mother often told me that I had a bad attitude. After years of consistently and frequently hearing this message, I no longer needed her to tell me there was something wrong with me. I told myself there must be something wrong with me.

I think the message many people get in our culture is: look good, fit in, do what everybody else does. There is enormous pressure to assimilate and conform. This way I was supposed to appear was inconsistent with my deeper values. I couldn't reconcile the two, my mind screamed out for help, and I think that's what the breakthrough was about.

Carla: Do you want to say anything more about your perspective on spiritual breakthroughs?

Lauren: Some providers will say that if you hear voices, you have a mental illness. When I ask young people, they say they hear voices every day and it is a deeply spiritual part of their identity; it is their way of talking with God.

I look back at what happened to me at 16, and I see it as immensely spiritual. There was a joining, a connection with a force greater than myself. It may have been my spirit; it may have been a Higher Power; it may have been my unconscious. It may have been all three coming together in a fiery blast that catapulted me to another dimension.

My "hallucinations" and "delusions" reflected areas of great pain and emptiness in my life. I used to think that every breath I took was a waste of oxygen and I didn't understand why I was alive. I felt powerless, unloved, unimportant and invisible. When my mind, informed by my heart and my spirit, bypassed the usual cognitive process and reached out for help, that's when the breakthrough happened. I suddenly felt powerful. I suddenly felt seen. I suddenly became important and felt loved. For the first time, I felt a strong sense of meaning, purpose, direction and capacity to focus and persevere.

As difficult as that journey was, I would not trade it for anything in the world. It has taught me about the mind's capacity to go to unknown depths and dimensions and to come out wiser and with a deeper sense of compassion and humanity.

But I've talked a lot… what do you think?

Carla: I don't remember any oppression from my own childhood that would have caused my mental illness. I had loving parents; my mom and my dad were very sensitive to my needs. I don't remember really having any feelings of oppression, so I can't agree with you in that aspect.

Lauren: Yes. That awareness took me by surprise. I didn't know that I was looking for a new understanding. I just thought this is the way life is and I put one foot in front of the other and I had a good job… but there was something missing.

Then I started hanging out with other people who had been through the mental health system. They had an understanding of ways our culture unintentionally harms us, different forms of sexism, racism, and what we call "mental health oppression." They started asking questions about my identity: *What do I love about being a woman and where does it get hard to be a woman? What do I love about being raised middle class and where does it get hard?* I learned more about how I got to be who I am.

I spent time with people who have a vision of a cooperative world that's inclusive and sensitive where we can celebrate our humanity and our individual difference. That's a very different world than what we have today.

Do you want to talk about your vision, what you want?

Carla: One thing I would change about the mental health system is that it doesn't focus on the whole person. What you get now is: *medication, more medication, and symptom control.*

My heart is really being drawn to creating a wellness center that is run by people who have personally experienced mental illness. I work in the mental health system now. Where I work we do have a good director, and we do try to bring out people's individual strengths, but I really want to create a center that is peer-run. That is my dream.

Lauren: Why is that important?

Carla: At a peer-run center we would be able to focus on recovery and on each individual's strengths — not just medication and case management and being told what to do. Ideally, all people would be able to go to a peer-run center where they can learn right away that they can make their own decisions and recover and see living examples of people who have done it.

It is a good thing that some people choose to work within the current mental health system and make changes from within, but I think my energy would be better spent building something different and unique other than what the system currently offers.

It's hard to go up against the system and work with people who have been in the system for so long and see themselves as powerless and their life is solely their mental illness. They come to the program all day, they go home to where people take care of them, and that's really all there is.

Lauren: Learned helplessness?

Carla: Yes. They learn helplessness through the mental health system.

Lauren: "Learned helplessness" is a phrase we can say, but for some people it's their whole life. They live in a group home where people tell them what to do and cook their meal.

Carla: Or they have families that over-function for them. That is the biggest mistake a family can make. It takes away a lot of an individual's power and self-esteem and self-confidence.

Lauren: How do families "over-function"?

Carla: As a family member, you can over-function for your loved ones by not letting them do what they can for themselves, making all of their decisions for them, and not allowing them to make their own mistakes. I am sure it is hard to watch a loved one make mistakes, but mistakes are how we learn. That is how everyone learns.

I know there may be times when someone going through a crisis needs more help, but as he or she gets better, you should step back. Sometimes you may even have to give the person a little nudge to get back in the driver's seat. I know my mom had to do that with me because I had lost faith in my abilities after coming out of the crisis.

Lauren: I think one the real disservices that our culture has done is to teach people to not trust their thinking and to depend on others. The greatest indignity the mental health system perpetuates is low expectations, reinforcing learned helplessness. I was taught that because something was wrong with me, my mind lacked the ability to come up with elegant solutions to challenges. I learned to give up my power, to not believe in myself. I saw myself as having limited ability and therefore limited worth.

Carla: I definitely agree that there's no room for individuality, especially in schools. All these children are put on medication to make them sit still in front of a desk for hours at a time.

Lauren: So kids are put on medication to make life easier for their teachers and perhaps for their parents? It's not that anything is necessarily wrong with them, but we teach them that something's wrong with them and then they internalize that and grow up believing something is wrong with them?

Carla: Yes, I see that. I can see where society does oppress children. They diagnose children with ADD and put them on Ritalin.

Lauren: So the labeling. . .

Carla: Starts young.

Lauren: It blames the individual instead of looking at the system.

Carla: It tells the child: *You have to have this pill because without it you don't have control over yourself.*

Lauren: You're powerless. That's a very dangerous message to tell a young person. It scares me. What are we doing to the brains of our children? What are we teaching them psychologically and emotionally?

I was talking to a young woman who was put on psych drugs at the age of eight.

She's off them now and she is doing fine today, but she said that it felt like she was underwater for many, many years. I try to imagine what it would feel like at 8, 9, or 10 to be underwater. When you're on medications, it can create this distance, this distortion of perception so that you're not quite with other people. You can't quite reach them and they can't reach you.

When I was put on medication at 16 I remember thinking, *There's something so wrong with my brain that they have to give me powerful drugs.* That was really scary, and I just internalized it all and believed it with every cell in my body. I believed that I was so damaged that I needed these drugs and I needed to be institutionalized.

Carla: As a society we overmedicate our children and expect everyone to conform. If I could run off and move to the mountains somewhere and home-school my children and isolate them from the evil in this world, I feel none of us would need medication – including me.

Lauren: We live in an insane world. Our culture is so obsessed with increasing productivity that sometimes we forget what it means to be human. We are training our children to fit into an oppressive society focused on increasing profits at all costs.

What are we doing to our children? What are we doing to our teachers that we put them in situations where they are absolutely overwhelmed? They've got 30 students in the class, and testing standards that are getting higher all the time. It's not manageable, so we drug our kids and give them the message they're powerless. We blame the individual instead of looking at the problem, which is the system.

Your question was: *What does it mean that mental illness can be learned?* I believe that if you are told something long enough and often enough, you come to believe it. Through schools and other institutions, we are told how to look, what to eat, what to wear, and how to behave if we want to be accepted into the mainstream of society. When I was young, I was taught that there was something wrong with me. I wasn't "normal." Well, maybe I don't want to be normal. Why be normal? I would rather work with others towards creating a peaceful, rational, cooperative, inclusive and just world.

What the system does now is blame the individual and it doesn't look at oppression. It doesn't look at how society and the system contributed to the development of what they call "mental illness."

I'm glad you said that you could see it, that you could see how that happens.

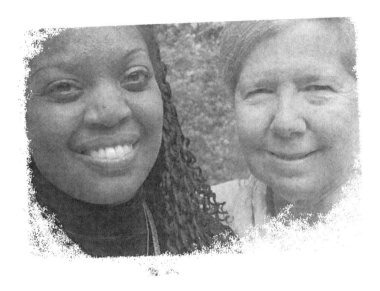

What does it mean when we say "people can recover from mental illness"?

Mitzi: Michelle, what is the most important part of your story of recovery?

Michelle: When a diamond is found in a cave, it's rough and rugged and ugly. You have to take a hammer and chisel and constantly work at it. It takes a long time to get that tiny little piece of diamond just the shape that you want it. The hardships are the chisel and the hammer. We're rough in the beginning, but once the chisel is done, you're that diamond.

Mitzi: Can you tell one thing that was a chisel and a hammer for you?

Michelle: I was in a car accident on April 11th, 1997, and I suffered a severe brain injury and that slowed me down just a little bit.

Mitzi: Don't be ridiculous, you're the least slowed-down person I ever saw.

Michelle: (laughing) I do a great job of covering it up. When I sit down to read a book, I'm a little bit slower in understanding what each sentence is saying. I have to take my time and kind of eat through each sentence. But that little bit of slowness makes it so that I can see things in other people. If you take the time to truly look at a person, you can catch the beauty in them. Everybody has beauty in them; nobody is without it.

Mitzi: How do you define mental health recovery for yourself? I think I've heard you say it in one sentence: The life you have now, as tough as it is, your regular everyday life is the one you want. How did you get from where you were to where you are now?

Michelle: I believe recovery is a choice. Even with mental health disabilities, we all still have the faculties to make a choice. You can either stay in the hospital and let somebody else take care of you and be dumbed-down by overmedication, or you can choose the life you want to lead, and work yourself toward it no matter how long it takes.

Mitzi: How did you apply the strength and courage to change?

Michelle: My WRAP (Wellness Recovery Action Plan) helped a lot. At the beginning, I would have to practice it every single day. I used to be the fight or the flight. With the flight, I'd disappear. I'd be out of the room. I could be on stage in the middle of getting ready to sing, and I'm gone. The fight is my mad-dog trigger. I'd start barking right back. Through using WRAP, I taught myself that if you look a person straight in the eye, you can make them back down no matter how angry they are without saying a single word. I look them in the face, I look them in the eye, stand tall, stand firm, look at them and then quietly tell them what's on my mind. It diffuses my mad-dog trigger and it helps diffuse the other person.

Mitzi: Tell me what WRAP is?

Michelle: It is a plan you create for your recovery. You lay out a daily maintenance schedule for yourself, you plan your wellness tools, you build up a support system, you take personal responsibility for your actions, you educate yourself about your disability, and you advocate for yourself. Hope is the foundation.

Mitzi: As a result of your recovery journey, have you uncovered previously unknown strengths or skills?

Michelle: I used to be agoraphobic. I stayed in my house the majority of the time for more than 10 years. Part of my recovery was starting to go to the vocational center, which got me around other people. It pulled me out of my world and into other people's worlds. The vocational center also sent me to a training to become a WRAP facilitator and lead groups.

They sat me down and said, "Michelle, you need to do this. This is exactly what fits you." That has given me direction for my life. It has given me a goal. I learned something I didn't know I could do: I can stand up and talk in front of people and encourage them. It gives me something to look forward to so that my depression doesn't go so dark and so deep and so heavy.

No matter how far we fall or how deep the depths of our mental illness, we can recover from it. We can come back from it. As a WRAP facilitator, I get opportunities to speak on a regular basis to my peers and to caseworkers about hope and recovery. I tell them: We can't just hope by ourselves. We need our supporters to have hope, too. Sometimes our supporters need to hold on to hope for us, so that we can gain back our hope when we lose it.

Mitzi: Is there anything that you cannot leave out in your recovery story? Is there anything where you feel: *Wait a minute! I've got to make sure this gets in there?*

Michelle: This is the part I left out in my story: When I was a kid, a family member would give me chocolate Ex-Lax as a candy reward. He would wake me up in the middle of the night and tell me how horrible it is to be fat. He was an alcoholic.

When my children were taken away, alcohol became my food all day and night – wine, mouthwash and sleeping pills. I could drink about four or five large bottles easily and still not sleep. I used diet pills during the day and sleeping pills at night. When I could not get wine or vodka, I turned to NyQuil and mouth wash. I was self-medicating to keep the mania under control and the depression at bay.

I almost died being under the delusion I could fly off a bridge. Alcohol is not the answer for dealing with mental health symptoms. I thought it helped me. It did not. It only brought me harm. Sometimes when I remember all I have lived through I am very tempted to have a drink, but my medication takes the edge off my disability, and I use meditation and prayer to help keep in control.

Now my work as a WRAP facilitator helps remind me why I am alive: to help others and to give of myself. I can't do that if I am depressed and drunk. Alcohol, diet pills, sleeping pills and Ex-Lax are no longer my gods.

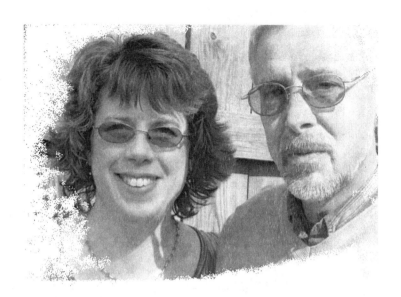

What's the difference between recovery and salvation?

Ken: Let me begin by asking you this: We use the word *recovery* in a very generic sense in the mental health field. What's the difference between *recovery* and *salvation?*

Debra: Wow, that's a tough question! The two have been so intertwined for me. Where I've walked more and more in faith, my recovery has gotten stronger. I know that a lot of people who go to church view mental illness as demonic, or as a character flaw or sin. I see it as biochemical; it just happens to be what I ended up with.

Ken: That's the chemist in you!

Debra: Yeah, it's the chemist in me! Because medications help me so much, I have to believe there is some chemical component for me. But there's an emotional component and a spiritual component as well. Once I'm on medication, I'm still not altogether normal. Sometimes I have noise in my head.

There have been a couple times when people have prayed over me – prayed about specific spirits – and suddenly all the noises cleared. I believe that there's a spiritual component to it for me. I believe in demons, and I believe in good and evil and spirits.

For a while I thought that I was letting God down. The Bible talks about being joyful in all circumstances and I thought, *I haven't figured out how to be joyful when I'm in the midst of depression.* I thought I was depressed because I was not doing something I'm supposed to be doing spiritually. Then I went on this church retreat and a lady who I didn't know came up to me and said, "I have a word from God for you and it makes no sense to me, but I'm just going to share it. God says that you're on the road he has for you. He showed me this road, and there are potholes – some of them are so deep that when you're in them, you can't see out. But it's the road you're supposed to be on."

That was the first time I started to see that depression might not be something that God was judging me for. I felt that God was there in the midst of the struggle with me. I felt he was saying, "I am with you and this is the road I have prepared for you. This is part of your life's path."

The Bible says that God is close to the brokenhearted and God is with those who are struggling and with those who are oppressed, but I really wasn't applying that to me. I had that quiet peace and contentment for the first time after that.

I hold on to the fact that God created me, He surely knows how messed up I am, and He loves me anyway. Jesus chose to hang out with people whose lives were a mess, so I figure I fit right in. He picked out the people who others judged, and he said, "Come, spend time with me." And the people who had all the money and all the power, those are the people that he scorned.

Ken: We grew up in a culture where everything is supposed to be perfect and sterile. When some people – especially people that work in the mental health field – see someone who is intense and real it scares the hell out of them. For a moment, they have to decide, "Do I accept my own anguish, or do I continue to block it out and play the game?" A lot of people just play the game.

Debra: I have trouble being around people who are like that.

Ken: Listen, my last hospitalization was in 1994. I was crying and crying and said, "I have to get back to the hospital and be around my people, people who can speak my language." I wanted to be around people who could acknowledge that they were suffering, that that is simply part of the human condition. Since that last time in the hospital, I've been able to find other people who have been real, so I haven't had to go back.

Debra: I've found a group of people in the church who are moving in that direction. In the church I'm involved in now, they talk about being transparent and acknowledging where your struggles are. Everybody has struggles. I've found that the Christian community is a place where, classically, people feel alone in their struggles, because you're supposed to be a "good Christian person."

Ken: This is an honest question. I've asked it many times: Do we do a disservice by not recognizing a higher power in the mental health field?

At our mental health agency we offer what we call "activities of daily living" and we don't offer spirituality. My belief is that this hinders people's recovery. There is a need within us as human beings for spirituality to ground us.

In Alcoholics Anonymous, one of the first steps is accepting a higher power and giving it a deified name. In the mental health field, we are very big into self-empowerment without any sense that there's a basic human need to have a relationship with something higher.

Debra: I think when you have a mental illness and go to the hospital, you're stripped of power and the power is given to other people. It's given to the psychiatrists and to the case managers and to the counselors. That's not the same as choosing to give up power and giving it to God. Empowerment is coming to trust yourself and taking back some of that power that you've given to other people when you don't need to give it to them anymore.

In the big picture and in the little details of life, God is in control. He is going to bring it together, and He is going to redeem the mistakes I make. All of it is in His hands, but I am still responsible. I still need to live out my life and do the things I need to do to recover. He has allowed me to know what some of those things are.

Suffering is not for nothing. It's not that God wants us to suffer because He's mean. Times of suffering are the times when we learn the most, we change the most, and we grow the most. I don't enjoy being in those times, but that's what has transformed my life: the different types of suffering, small or large, that I've gone through. That's what caused me to be uncomfortable enough to need to change, and grow, and adapt. I became a better person because I got uncomfortable.

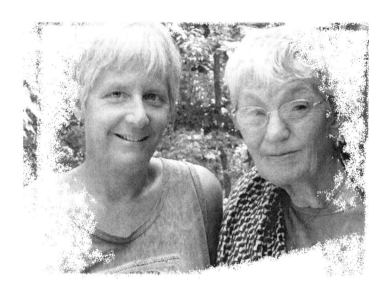

What happens when you give power to "crazy people"?

Bev: How do you envision the mental health advocacy movement helping those who have been labeled with mental illness?

Lauren: It's hard for someone who hasn't been locked up in a seclusion room and on heavy doses of psychiatric medication to understand what it's like. Among people who have been through the system, there's a *simpático* way we understand each other.

There's just nothing like being with someone who can hold your hand and say, "I've been there; you're not alone and you can recover; your dreams can come true. There are many other people who have been through what you've gone through and they are able to have a full life."

A lot of us have gone through this and we know what helped us go beyond surviving to thriving. Most of what I've learned about my own recovery journey has been from people who have freed themselves from the damage that the mental health system inflicts. People with the experience of mental health recovery know what works and what doesn't. We need to see more people with this lived experience leading the way. We need to be central in all the decisions that are being made that affect us.

It's scary for the system to give up some of their power to us "crazy people."

Bev: I've been in Virginia about nine years and I am extremely grateful for the opportunity to be in the mental health recovery movement. But when I go back to my native state, my friends from the mental health center don't have the slightest notion that a recovery approach to mental health services is possible. Where do we go from here?

Lauren: I don't think there's any more powerful way we can communicate how far we can go than through our own experiences. We can be the wind under each other's wings.

I didn't have the insight to understand the importance of boldly saying, "I was labeled with chronic schizophrenia but it's not who I am." Then, when the White House New Freedom Commission on Mental Health was formed in 2003, I saw that the President had appointed someone who had a diagnosis of schizophrenia and who was also a psychiatrist. It gave me courage and motivated me to come out publicly as a psychiatric survivor.

Bev: I was once in an art therapy group in a mental health center, and I happened to know that the therapist had been in a psychiatric hospital, but she was not disclosing. It made me angry because at the time I was really feeling the stigma of being labeled. Years later, I heard that she had come out and disclosed. In my mind, it was an acknowledgement that she understood where we were coming from.

Lauren: People who have been labeled with mental illness are increasingly realizing that there is power in numbers and that when we do come together our voice is stronger. The disability rights motto is: *Nothing about us without us.*

Bev: After the tragedy at Virginia Tech, the media reported that the shooter had received mental health services. Do you see a noticeable difference in the mental health system following this incident?

Lauren: Yes, after Virginia Tech the mental health laws changed. Rather than giving people what they need, now there's more use of coercion. A lot more money is being allocated into force. It makes me very angry. It's the complete opposite of what is needed, and now there's less money available for what really works.

The media's reaction has been fueling fire. There has been an increase of fear and discrimination against people labeled with mental illness. It's understandable that people are afraid. We all want to be safe. We get scared and our thinking gets a little narrow and we just want *those people* away from us… so lock them up or force them into treatment, even if it's not effective or makes things worse. The use of the word *treatment* here is inappropriate. It is really *coercion* – a violation of civil rights.

These changes in the law are not helpful, they do more damage, and they have the opposite effect: They scare people away from the mental health system. Now people are afraid of being honest for fear of being locked up against their will. People don't feel safe in a society that treats them as less than human, so they go into hiding. Instead of reaching out for help, people hold it in until one day it'll explode like we saw at Virginia Tech. What happened at Virginia Tech will happen again.

Bev: Are you aware of any extraordinarily helpful measures that are taking place across the country?

Lauren: There are many islands of hope and pockets of empowerment. There are organizations run by people who have been labeled with mental illness all across Virginia and all across the country. They are doing amazing work: training, advocacy, education, and alternatives to hospitalization. These are places where we serve as role models for each other. For example, Rose House in New York City is an alternative to hospitalization. People thrive there and do well afterwards. It costs 1/10th of the traditional system.

People are creating communities that are empowering, inclusive, and integrated into society. We're working collaboratively; stepping over hurdles; writing by-laws; developing Boards of Directors; getting incorporated; renting spaces; and starting wellness centers.

When we're given money and power and people get out of the way, miracles happen.

Bev: You've talked about swings between eating too much and eating too little or sleeping too much and sleeping too little. How do you go about maintaining balance at such times? Or is it just a part of who you are and how you operate?

Lauren: Maybe maintaining balance is oversold. Maybe I want to explore other dimensions of myself I don't even know about yet. What's so great about balance? When I have huge challenge in front of me that's very stressful, I'm reaching deeper inside myself to find new thinking or a new level of courage to speak my truth. Sometimes I'll eat less or sleep less because I'm so focused on writing a grant or preparing a speech. Providers or family members might get nervous and say, "Oh, that's too much; that's too stressful; you don't want to lose your balance."

I've worked as a professional in the mental health field for over 25 years. I get nervous; I get anxious; I have self-doubt; I get excited; I have a vision of a world that's very different than our current culture. Sometimes I sleep too much; sometimes I eat too much; sometimes I'm tired and don't have a lot of energy. So if people want to label that as "mental illness" or "symptoms" they are certainly free to do that, but I think that label diminishes our humanity.

How do we reach new highs or accomplishments if we're so focused on staying balanced and keeping a status quo – a stasis in our own energy? Certainly we want a certain amount of balance, but life is not about balance all the time. It's about stretching and that means taking risks. I am learning to grow beyond perceived limitations.

I'm not talking about anything too wild or dangerous, but I do want to experience life while I'm living.

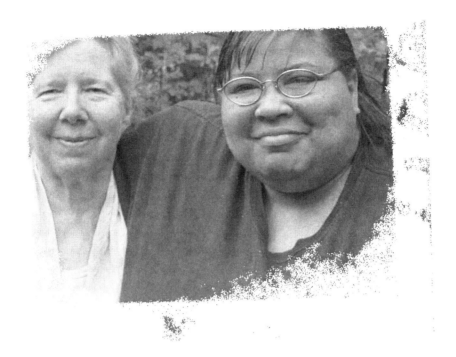

What is the hardest thing to get people to understand about mental illness?

Mitzi: What is the biggest challenge in helping people understand mental illness?

Myra: The biggest thing is the way people discriminate against you, treat you differently, and shun you. At Virginia Tech, a student who had a psychiatric diagnosis took lives of 32 students, plus himself. This just reinforced every negative image that's ever been put on TV about mental illness. People who were closed-minded thought, *Aha! I knew it! I told you!* The media already portrayed people with mental illness as violent and dangerous. The fact is this: A person who has a mental illness is more likely to be a victim of crime than a perpetrator.

I try to change one mind at a time. I don't have the resources to go up against the media, but I have the resources to challenge the next door neighbor who tells me an off-color joke about somebody being crazy.

I think when you deal with stigma you have to pick and choose. If you attacked stigma every time it attacked you, it would tire you out. That's what you'd be doing all day long. I make it a point when I meet new people and new employers to give some time for them to try to get to know me as a person before I disclose that I struggle with mental health issues. Sometimes it works. Sometimes it doesn't work.

Mitzi: Can you tell me about a time when you experienced stigma?

Myra: When I started getting jobs, it was terrible. I remember one time I went to a psychiatric hospital and when I got back to work my supervisors said they needed a letter from my doctor stating I was safe to work with children – even though I had gotten glowing results on my work evaluation. If I were to know then everything I know now, I would have been able to better advocate for myself.

Mitzi: How would you have fought the way you were treated there?

Myra: Well, I probably would have reviewed the Americans with Disabilities Act and made sure that they weren't requesting anything that was unreasonable. I probably would have consulted with somebody from Legal Aid to make sure my rights were protected as a person who has a disability. I probably wouldn't have been so intimidated and given in so easily to every request.

Mitzi: You said that you believe children with mental health problems are treated differently than adults?

Myra: I've had mental health problems since I was a child. When people look at a child with problems, they pity that child. "Poor child, something must have happened to her." When people look at an adult with mental health problems, they are quick to judge.

I'll give you an example. At the mental health program where I work, a lot of members have hygiene problems and this rubs some staff the wrong way. Not me. I don't say a word. I know what it feels like to wake up in the morning and not feel like doing anything, including getting in the shower. I know how it feels to lay in bed for days and do nothing.

So guess what? The people at our program are one step ahead of me. They got out of the house this morning. I would have still been in bed. Some staff members don't realize the effort that it takes to just get up and get out; if they did they wouldn't say anything about the hygiene issue. They wouldn't be so appalled. I have nothing but empathy and understanding for people in that place. So when I see someone I say, "Hello, I'm glad to see you. How can I help you today? What can I do?"

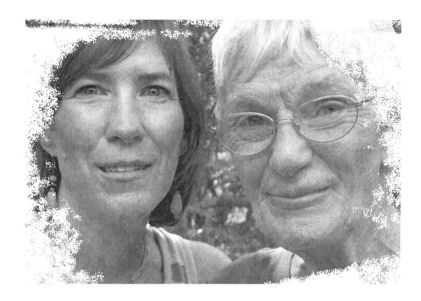

Bev: Carla, what is the hardest thing to get people to understand about mental illness?

Carla: That you can be a good parent. During my psychosis, I took care of my children very well. Even though I had all of these ideas in my head about things going on, I still fixed their meals and did all the things with them that I was doing before. Some people think if you're psychotic you can't function. That is a misunderstanding. Right after I started taking anti-psychotic medication, I needed assistance because I felt surreal and disconnected and just could not stay awake because of the side effects. When I found the right medication and dosage, I was able to take back full responsibility for my children.

Bev: How do you deal with mental health stigma and discrimination?

Carla: Changing people's preconceived ideas about mental illness is a big passion of mine. Stigma is what kept my family from getting my brother the help that he needed. It also kept us from healing after his suicide.

I try to fight stigma whenever I get the chance. I've told my story at seminars and to the Hanover County Police Department. I advised them on how to deal with somebody in psychosis: Stay calm and don't overreact. I spoke at the state psychiatric hospital near where I live. I shared my story in an article in a Richmond newspaper. That was all part of my effort to reduce stigma and say, "Hey, look, I'm a part of this community. I'm a loving mother, wife, daughter, friend and neighbor."

There's a song called "Psycho" performed by Puddle of Mudd. The lyrics are "I'm a schizophrenic psycho. I'm a paranoid flake." I wrote the radio station and record label a long letter saying, "Yes, I have been diagnosed with schizophrenia, but I am not a psycho or a paranoid flake." It makes me so angry that these songs are being listened to by college children where there's so much stigma already. College-aged people who happen to have been labeled with mental illness have a very rough road.

I think *Firewalkers* will give another viewpoint. We hope a cultural change will take place in how people view mental illness.

Debra: Tracy, how do you deal with people who are caught in stigma and don't understand?

Tracy: When people are very hardened about mental illness, what I do is this: I show them. I show them in action what kind of person I am. When they see I can manage something that means maybe others like me could manage something, too.

People who don't deal with mental illness on a daily basis still have times when they have mental heartbreak because of a specific situation or circumstance. Everybody gets a taste of it. Everybody doesn't know what it's like to be diabetic, but everybody knows what it's like to have mental illness.

I also know that there are some people who will never change. Sometimes I get really paranoid: *What are they thinking? What are they saying? How are they going to label me?* I'm almost 50 and I've come to realize it really doesn't matter. In the past, I've been very secretive because of stigma and worrying what people will think. But people know if you have something to deal with and you're trying to hide it. They'll figure it out.

Debra: Especially once you put it in a book.

Tracy: (laughs) Yes, and I'm really apprehensive about having my story in this book, are you?

Debra: Everyone knows I have mental health struggles. I don't hide it too much. I'm actually nervous about my parents because they *know,* but in my family you don't talk about such things, and you certainly don't put it in a book!

Debra: My mom and dad probably won't talk about it to me. My brother will probably say, "Are you crazy?" And I'll say, "Yes, and I have the papers to prove it!"

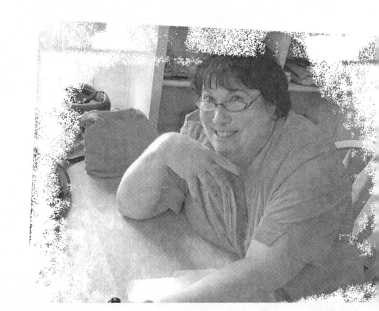

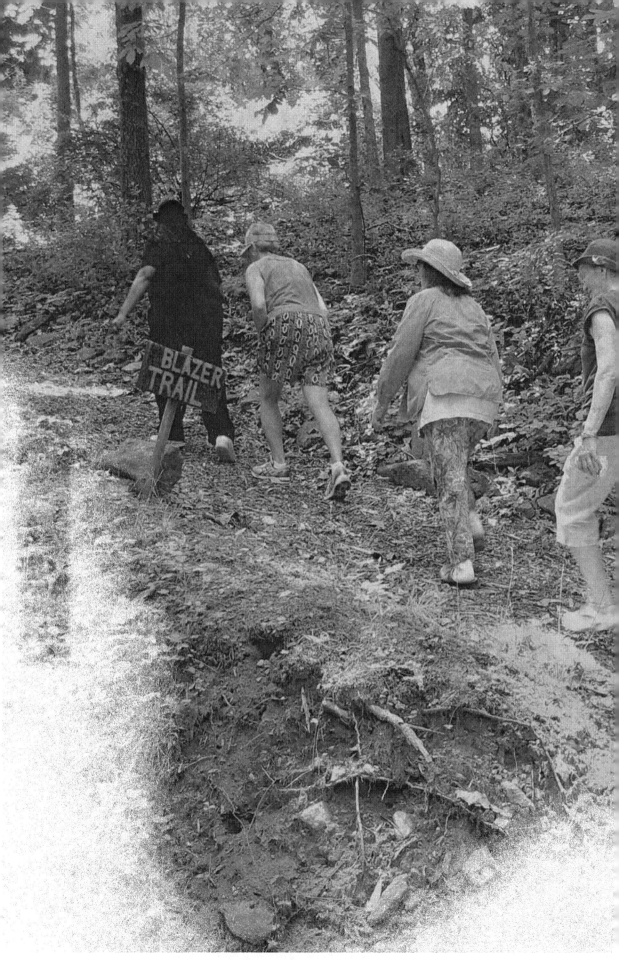

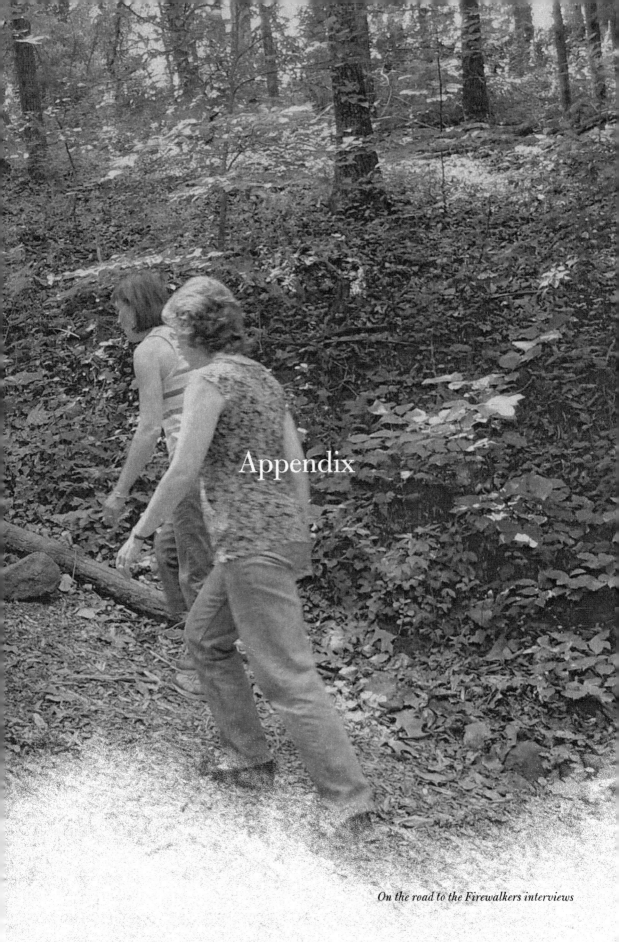

Appendix

On the road to the Firewalkers interviews

Firewalkers Editorial Team

Bev Ball

Bev is grateful that her experience with mental illness has brought her opportunities – including mental health leadership training, participating on VOCAL's Board of Directors, leadership roles at a local peer-run mental health center, serving as a Mental Health Planning Council representative to national conferences, and helping create an Emotional Wellness Ministry at her church. Her recent fun projects have been live poetry, folk music and dance performance. Bev hopes that the Firewalkers Project will kindle within each individual an awareness of how unfortunate circumstances can spark new opportunities.

This is my 72nd year. I've had over 50 years of dealing with mental illness. I will not forget. My personal prediction was that I would spend the rest of my life in the hospital—with the linoleum floors, the day room, and the TV. Not pleasant. Becoming part of the mental health recovery movement and part of VOCAL has been enriching and satisfying. I believe that if well-written, every single person's story could be a best seller.

Ann Benner

Ann is the Program Director of the VOCAL Network, a student, a mother, a social worker, and an artist.

I want the world to understand that people with mental health struggles are to be respected and honored for the extra work they constantly do to function in the world. I want people who are newly diagnosed to respect and honor the growth opportunity they have been given. It is the chance to understand and accept humanity and the spirit with far greater depth. But Firewalkers is not a laurel — it is an attitude of awareness, openness and humility.

Debra Knighton

Being in and out of the hospital... this experience guided my vocation and the fact that I met my husband and have kids. It not only made me a more compassionate, understanding person, but it's done that for my parents, husband, and kids. My kids are growing up with a very different world view than I did.

Having had the opportunity to be intimately involved in the creation of such a powerful book has been a tremendous blessing for me. I have been touched by the way the peer editorial team has held each story (including my own) with such respect and gentleness. What a gift to have been part of this team through the whole editorial process.

Yolande Long

Yolande is a social worker who works for the VOCAL Network as the Communications and Events Coordinator. She is happily married with three children – most of whom are fully grown but still keep her on her toes – and a beautiful granddaughter who continually teaches her what life and love is really all about.

I grew up with an older brother who dealt with serious mental illness. There was no mental health "recovery movement" that could offer him hope for his future. His illness was frightening to our family and to our small community, as his behavior was erratic. There was a lot of stigma attached; some people acted as though if they got too close to him or us they could catch it. As a child experiencing all that, I grew up frightened that I might one day be diagnosed with mental illness myself. I associated it with something terrifying and isolating.

*As life sometimes goes, **I was** diagnosed with a mental illness when I was a late teen – but I had experienced the symptoms of it since the age of 10 without knowing what it was or how to get help. I despaired that I would never completely well. I spent most of my energy hiding it, and my day-to-day life was exhausting beyond measure.*

Then I met someone who had the same disorder, and she offered me hope that I could be well. She introduced me to someone else who gave me more hope! Before I knew it, I found all these people who were dealing with mental illness – just like me – and they were wise and funny and good and kind and creative and living lives that were meaningful! They weren't hiding, because they'd found a community where they didn't have to – a community of hope and recovery that values us for who we are, accepts us because of our life experiences, and encourages us to become more. All of this came to me because of that diagnosis!

So now I know how blessed I am to be living this life and to have walked through the fire. And I know how privileged I am to have helped in some small part with this amazing book.

Ken Moore

Life can be incredibly difficult. It's not surprising to me that I went stark raving mad. The question I ask myself is, "Why did these other people not go mad?" When the values we have are not lived out in our culture, how do people not find themselves with some form of profound dissonance? The beauty of and the miracle is that people who honestly search for answers to these questions are recovering. And doing it in a significant way.

Robert Johnson, a Jungian Psychologist, once said, "We are born unconsciously whole, we become consciously shattered, and the challenge then in life is to become consciously whole." That's the challenge we face when we have a serious mental illness — how to move beyond the shattering towards recovery and becoming whole.

For some people just learning about recovery can be a revelation—a guiding light — a composition of hope. The more this revelation happens, the less impossible recovery appears. A person develops a mental illness for whatever reason. The real journey, task, and challenge is to recover.

There are a few moments in each of our lives that hold such important meaning that they draw us into a greater magnitude of spiritual clarity. These moments, events, and pursuits are what increase consciousness. The Firewalkers Project has been one of these defining moments in my life, giving me greater understanding and insight into what it means to recover.

Cassandra Nudel

Cassandra is a writer, educator, social justice advocate, and nonprofit consultant. Cassandra's work in mental health and disability rights began after her own experience of being homebound for 5 years, while living in solitude in a rural area. She is the project leader for the *Firewalkers* book and co-creator of several nonprofit grassroots mental health programs. Cassandra lives in Charlottesville, Virginia, where she enjoys sufi dancing, shamanism, organic cooking, dreamwork, sleeping, and playing with her cats, her sweetheart, and other loved ones.

*One day years ago, when I was living in solitude on the mountain, I read a book called **No Pity**, the story of the disability civil rights movement. The moment I opened it, something shifted in me. I stopped seeing myself as a lone traveler, a solitary black bird, whose life had taken a strange turn, and started seeing myself as part of a larger movement of people with disabilities. I started calling myself a person with disabilities. And felt proud of it.*

I didn't know it then, but of all this was leading me, slowly and circuitously, to where I am now – in a world filled with other people and part of creating a *mental health disability rights movement in Virginia. That day and that book changed me for good. My deepest hope for **Firewalkers** is that someday somewhere someone will pick up this book and feel what I felt then.*

Brian Parrish

Brian Parrish is a mental health activist and the Executive Director of VO-CAL. Brian is also a member of the Virginia Mental Health Planning Council and the System Leadership Council. Previously, he worked as the Program Director for the VOCAL CO-OP, a collective of peer-run mental health programs, and as a Peer Supporter at On Our Own of Charlottesville, a mental health recovery center.

***Firewalkers** is the story of how walking through the crucible of what is called mental illness, we have grown as people. It is a rough road, but we can become stronger and find a place within ourselves that is more powerful and deeper. It is about being broken open, being buried alive, being lost in the void, thrown into the lonely reaches of outer space. The question is: At the end of it when you step out of the fire, are you still whole, and how have you changed?*

Malaina Poore

Malaina lives in an enchanted cottage in a holler with her two whirlwind children and makes personal art whenever she gets the chance. Her current passion is in finding ways to combine art, activism and community.

***Firewalkers** is not an outsider's viewpoint, not an anthropologist's perspective. Everybody on the editorial team has shared similar experiences. My life has been shaped by my inner emotional world; it's a passionate one. I've had times when I felt completely hopeless and I felt I was so unique in my hopelessness. I never feel that way anymore.*

I loved reading Debra's story and hearing her say: I can be grouchy at times and need people to hang in there with me, and in turn, I will hang in there with others. Sometimes I wonder what's going on with other people and it so helpful to have seven people explain it honestly.

Cynthia Power

Part of what fires do is effect chemical change that can't be reversed. The recovery movement is so exciting to me. As a person with a long-term psychiatric label, *my current theme is balance. The **Firewalkers** gathering and interviews were exceptionally special for me. It gave me so much that I'm feeling teary. I knew it was great, but I didn't know it was going to do this to me.*

Mitzi Ware

Mitzi Ware is a social worker who lives in Charlottesville with her wonderful husband, dog and cat. She especially enjoys reading, knitting, doing numerous art projects, playing the piano, singing, biking and hanging out with close friends.

*I remember walking on the downtown mall and catching the cover of the newly-released book **Girl, Interrupted** in the window of the Williams Corner Bookstore. I knew it was my book and promptly went in and bought it. That book and **The Unquiet Mind** had a huge impact on me. From them I learned that you could recover from mental illness. This was new. You could live a happy, productive life. This was new, too. It had been a lonely and secretive journey through several psychiatrists' offices. Then one day a therapist commented to me that the psychiatric establishment sees through the lens of pathology – why not look at your situation from the standpoint of health and recovery? My work with her, and reading other books about recovery, provided a major turning point for me. Working on the **Firewalkers** project has been a wonderful, nurturing experience.*

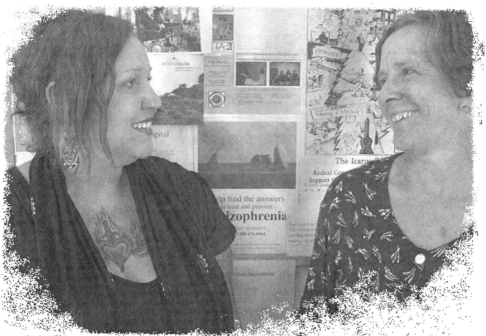

Ann & Malaina

Firewalkers Glossary

*Key Terms and Important Resources
from the Firewalkers Interviews*

Mental Health Conferences

Conferences are places where you can connect with peers and learn about mental health self-determination and recovery. *Nationally:* The Alternatives Conference is organized by and for people with psychiatric labels. This conference offers in-depth assistance on peer-delivered services and self-help methods, as well as a rich social, artistic, and healing environment. *In Virginia:* The VOCAL Conference is a three-day conference for mental health peers held every year in the Spring by the VOCAL Network. 877-862-5638. **www.vocalvirginia. org** (click on "About Us" tab and choose the Vocal Network).

Mental Health Leadership Academy

Consumer Empowerment Leadership Training (CELT) is a free 3-day training that teaches leadership skills to people who have been diagnosed with mental illness. *In Virginia:* 804-257-5591. **www.mhav.org** *Nationally:* Similar leadership academies exist in other states. Contact your statewide mental health consumer association or one of the national centers listed at the end of this section. A list of statewide associations can be found at **www.ncmhcso.org/ members.htm**

Mental Illness & Violence

It is a myth that people with mental illness are dangerous and should be feared. Studies show that people with mental illness are more likely to be victims of violence than perpetrators of violence. We are no more violent than the general

population. *Violence and Mental Illness: The Facts.* <u>www.stopstigma.samhsa.</u>
<u>gov</u> 800-540-0320.

Mental Illness & Mortality

A recent study shows that people with serious mental illness served by our
public mental health system die, on average, at least 25 years earlier than the
general population. Many people who have been diagnosed with mental illness
and their allies are using this information as inspiration and motivation to call
for reform in the mental health system. *Morbidity & Mortality in People with
Serious Mental Illness.* <u>www.nasmhpd.org</u>

NAMI Family-to-Family Classes

The NAMI Family-to-Family Education Program is a free, 12-week course
for family caregivers of individuals with severe mental illnesses. The course is
taught by trained family members. <u>www.nami.org</u> 800-950-6264

National Coalition

The National Coalition of Mental Health Consumer/Survivor Organizations is
designed to ensure that mental health consumer/survivors have a major voice
in the development and implementation of health care, mental health, and
social policies at the state and national levels, empowering people to recover
and lead a full life in the community. Lauren Spiro, who is featured in this
book, is the Public Policy Director of this organization. <u>www.ncmhcso.org</u>
877-246-9058

Peer-run Programs

Peer-run Programs (also known as "consumer-run programs") are grassroots,
self-help programs led by people in recovery from mental illness. At a peer-run
program, the Board of Directors and staff would be all or mostly people who
have been diagnosed with mental illness. Peer-run programs include drop-
in center, employment centers, recovery groups, and more. To find a peer-
run program near you: *Nationally:* <u>www.cdsdirectory.org</u>, 800-553-4539.
In Virginia: <u>www.vocalvirginia.org</u>, (click on peer programs tab), 434-
243-7878. To create a new peer-run program or strengthen your existing program: See <u>www.vocalvirginia.org</u> (click on peer programs tab) for listings of
tools, resources, publications and trainings to help you get started.

Peer Support Specialists

Peer Support Specialists are people recovering from mental illnesses who use their experiences to help others. Peer Specialists are often employed within the mental health system. To learn more about peer specialists: **www.naops.org** 616-676-9230. To get trained to be a peer specialist (some programs are free or include scholarships) *In Virginia:* Virginia Human Services Training 434-970-2148; Recovery Innovations of Virginia 757-361-0255 **www.recoveryinnovations.org**; Virginia DMHMRSAS 804-786-9143. *Nationally:* **www.peersupport.org** 800 826-3632 and **www.dbsalliance.org** and **www.mentalhealthpeers.com.**

Recovery

What is mental health recovery? Recently, 110 people got together to answer this question. Participants included people diagnosed with mental illness, family members, providers, advocates, researchers, academicians, and public officials. This is the definition they came up with: "Mental health recovery is a journey of healing and transformation enabling a person with a mental health problem to live a meaningful life in a community of his or her choice while striving to achieve his or her full potential." *National Consensus Statement of Mental Health Recovery* **http://mentalhealth.samhsa.gov/publications/all-pubs/sma05-4129/**

Stigma & Discrimination

You can find resources about combating stigma and tools to help in the recovery process at **www.whatadifference.samhsa.gov** and **www.promoteacceptance.samhsa.gov.** We also recommend the book *Don't Call Me Nuts: Coping with the Stigma of Mental Illness* by Patrick Corrigan and Robert Lundin.

VOCAL

Founded and run by people who have been diagnosed with mental illness, VOCAL works to connect people to people and to improve Virginia's mental health services. We promote mental health recovery, empowerment, self-determination and peer leadership. VOCAL is the organization that made this *Firewalkers* book. **www.vocalvirginia.org** 434-243-7878

WRAP

Wellness Recovery Action Plan (WRAP) was developed by Mary Ellen Copeland and a group of people who experience mental health difficulties. These people learned that they can identify what makes them well and then use their own wellness tools to relieve difficult feelings and maintain wellness. The result has been recovery and long-term stability. Your WRAP program is designed by you in practical, day-to-day terms and holds the key to getting and staying well. To learn more about WRAP: www.mentalhealthrecovery.com. 802-254-2092. To train to become a WRAP facilitator (some programs are free or include scholarships) *Nationally:* www.mentalhealthrecovery.com. 802-254-2092. *Virginia:* www.vocalvirginia.org (click on the "About Us" tab and choose the REACH program) or call 757-618-1650.

Looking for something else?

If you'd like to learn more about the mental health movement, recovery, self-determination, becoming a mental health advocate or any of the topics listed above we encourage you to contact these three national centers (all three are run by people who have been diagnosed with mental illness):

Depression and Bipolar Support Alliance (DBSA)

www.dbsalliance.org

National Empowerment Center

www.power2u.org

National Mental Health Consumers' Self-help Clearinghouse

www.mhselfhelp.org

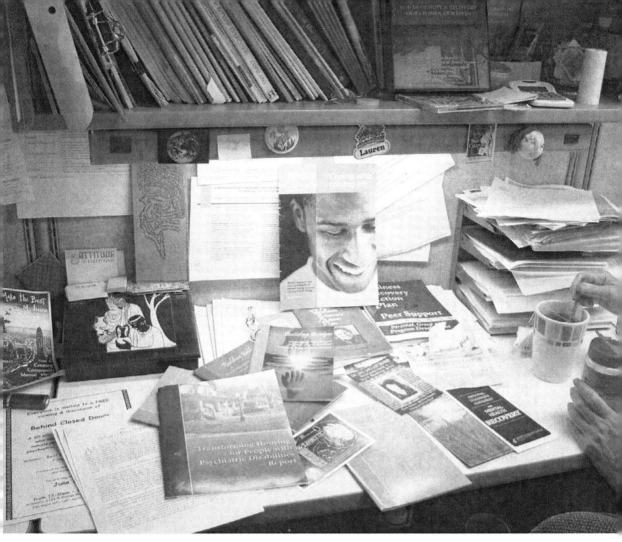

Lauren's desk at work

Books that Changed
(or Saved) Our Lives

from the Firewalkers storytellers & editorial team

An Unquiet Mind: A Memoir of Moods and Madness by Kay Redfield Jamison

Dr. Kay Redfield Jamison may be the foremost authority on manic-depressive illness. She is also one of its survivors. And it is this dual perspective—as healer and healed — that makes Jamison's memoir so lucid, learned, and profoundly affecting.

No Pity: People with Disabilities Forging a New Civil Rights Movement by Joseph Shapiro

A vibrant and compelling account of our century's last great civil rights movement. Over the last 30 years, disabled Americans have fought for freedom from the discrimination and oppression of medical, psychological, and bureaucratic establishments. This is the first popular history of the disability rights movement.

Spiritual Emergency by Stanislav Grof

Spiritual experience can feel like bliss, but it can also feel like hell. It can cause hallucinations, seizures, pain, panic attacks, mania, severe depression—all the symptoms of physical and mental illness. When people suffer this way, they may feel like they're going crazy, and their doctors may agree. The authors of this book think that in many cases, such a diagnosis is mistaken. They urge the adoption of a new category of clinical diagnosis, "spiritual emergency."

The Icarus Project: Navigating the Space Between Brilliance & Madness

About the Icarus Project: "We are a network of people living with experiences that are commonly labeled as bipolar or other psychiatric conditions. We believe we have mad gifts to be cultivated and taken care of, rather than diseases or disorders to be suppressed or eliminated." The term "mad gifts" which is used in this book comes from the Icarus Project. The Icarus website has many excellent guidebooks and materials including: *Friends Make the Best Medicine:* a guide to creating community mental health support networks, and *The Harm Reduction Guide to Coming Off of Psychiatric Drugs.* **http:// theicarusproject.net/**

Bricks & Dreams

Guidebooks from VOCAL show you how to create and grow your own grassroots mental health program. Our guidebooks include: *The Grant Seeker's Treasure Map & Orienteering Guide, Bricks & Dreams: A Transformation Guide to Peer-Run Programs, Blueprints for Change: How to Create a New Program, Fear of Filing: How to Become a 501c3 Nonprofit,* and many more tools and resources. Our email newsletter includes visionary ideas, key job openings, program updates, scholarship opportunities, and other tidbits and treasures for mental health advocates. **www.vocalsupportcenter.org**

Peace from Nervous Suffering & Hope and Help for Your Nerves
by Claire Weekes

This work offers help to those suffering from the commonest kind of nervous illness—the anxiety state (often called nervous breakdown). In addition, it offers advice to those whose illness is dominated by a particular fear—agoraphobia.

When Things Fall Apart by Pema Chodron

Drawn from traditional Buddhist wisdom, Pema Chodron's radical and compassionate advice for what to do when things fall apart in our lives goes against the grain of our usual habits and expectations. There is only one approach to suffering, Pema teaches, and that approach involves moving toward painful situations with friendliness and curiosity, relaxing into the essential groundlessness of our entire situation. It is there, in the midst of chaos, that we can discover the truth and love that are indestructible.

The Power of Positive Thinking by Norman Vincent Peale

Helps the reader achieve a happy, satisfying, and worthwhile life. With the practical techniques outlined in this book, you can energize your life—and give yourself the initiative needed to carry out your ambitions and hopes.

A Brilliant Madness by Patty Duke

Patty Duke addresses her struggle with manic-depressive disorder. From what it's like to live with manic-depressive disorder to the latest findings on its most effective treatments, this book provides insight into the challenge of mental illness and offers hope for all those who suffer from mood disorders and those who love and care for them.

The Language of Letting Go by Melody Beattie

Melody Beattie integrates her own life experiences and fundamental recovery reflections in this unique daily meditation book written especially for those who struggle with the issue of codependency. According to Beattie, "problems are made to be solved, and the best thing we can do is take responsibility for our own pain and self-care." Daily meditations remind readers that each day is an opportunity for growth and renewal.

Girl, Interrupted by Susanna Kaysen

A memoir of a young woman's two-year stay in a psychiatric hospital. This is a clearly written episodic account which challenges much conventional thinking about what is normal and what is deviant; what is sane and what is insane; and what is mental illness and what is recovery.

Spiritual Texts

Conversations with God by Neale Donald Walsch;
The Prophet by Khalil Gibran;
Books by Jiddu Krishnamurti;
Psalm 40, 42, 57: 1-2 from the Bible
(*King David does such a wonderful job of expressing what it's like to struggle with depression all the while looking to God for hope and help. – Debra*)

Please support your independent booksellers. If there are no independent booksellers in your area, these books can be ordered through VOCAL's bookstore affiliate program, www.vocalsafelink.org/astore.

Where to Share Your Story

Since we began the Firewalkers project, many people have contacted us with interesting and amazing stories they would like to share with the world. If you would like to share your story of your mental health journey, here are a few organizations you can contact.

National Empowerment Center Recovery Stories. Dedicated to the stories of folks who have had an experience of severe emotional anguish some call "mental illness" and who have had the experience of recovery. recoverystories@power2u.org. **www.power2u.org**

Mental Health America. Invites people with mental illnesses to break the silence and share their stories. Through real stories, others may find help and can open the door to the truth about mental illness. **www.mentalhealthamerica.net/real-lives**, 703-684-7722

Time to Change. Inspiring stories from people who have challenged mental health discrimination. If you have taken steps to raise awareness about mental health issues, this project can support you to tell your story in your own words. **http://time-to-change.org.uk/experiences-views/your-stories**

Stories of Self Determination. This blog is a place for people with disabilities to write stories about their lives. It is a place where you can write about what you did to get the life you wanted. You can also write about what kind of life you are trying to get, but don't have yet. http://selfdetermination.wordpress.com

Open Minds Quarterly is a literary magazine that publishes writing of consumers and survivors of mental illness: strong, creative, intelligent, human writers, people who have stories to share. Our magazine opens minds, and opens hearts. 705-675-9193, xt. 8286 http://nisa.on.ca *(click on the link for Open Minds Quarterly)*

VOCAL Network – Welcomes poems, stories and personal writing by mental health peers who live in Virginia. Send your writing to network@vocalvirginia. org. Please include a note indicating that you are giving permission to publish this piece. 877-862-5638

The MindFreedom Personal Story Project collects histories from psychiatric survivors and mental health consumers about their experiences of survival, resistance, recovery and self-determination in the mental health system. www.mindfreedom.org, 877-MAD-PRID

StoryCorps. Honor and celebrate one another's lives through listening. Almost 30,000 everyday people have shared life stories with family and friends in our StoryBooths. Millions listen to their broadcasts on public radio and the web. One of the largest oral history projects of its kind. www.storycorps.net

In Our Own Voice (IOOV) is a unique public education program developed by NAMI, in which trained speakers share compelling personal stories about living with mental illness and achieving recovery. www.nami.org. 703-524-7600

Firewalkers
Funders & Supporters

Firewalkers is made possible thanks to support from:

National Consumer Survivor Technical Assistance Center (NCSTAC)

The purpose of NCSTAC, a program of Mental Health America (**www.mental-healthamerica.net**), is to strengthen consumer organizations by providing technical assistance in the form of research, informational materials, and financial aid. Learn more at **www.ncstac.org**

The Virginia Department of Behavioral Health and Developmental Services

Available to citizens statewide, Virginia's public mental health, intellectual disability and substance abuse services system is comprised of 16 state facilities and 40 locally-run community services boards, which serve children and adults who have or who are at risk of mental illness, serious emotional disturbance, intellectual disabilities, or substance use disorders. Learn more at: **http://www.dmhmrsas.virginia.gov/OMH-default.htm**

Campaign for Mental Health Recovery

This book was made possible through funding from the Substance and Mental Health Services Administration Center for Mental Health Services as part of the national Campaign for Mental Health Recovery—a national public education effort that improves the general understanding of mental illness, promotes recovery, and encourages help-seeking behaviors across the age span. To learn more visit: **http://www.stopstigma.samhsa.gov** and **http://www.whatadifference.org**. This campaign publishes and distributes myths and facts about mental illness:

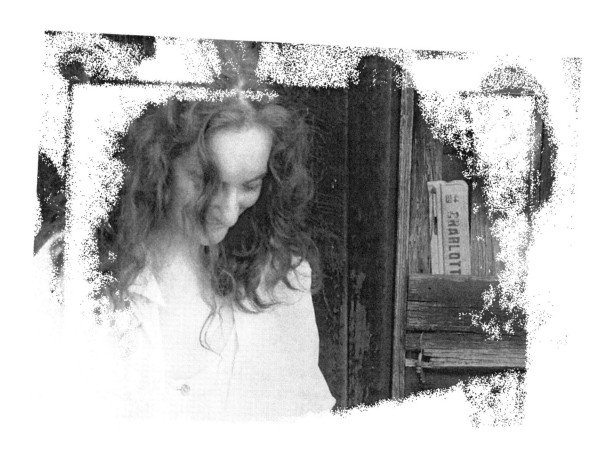

After the Fire

Editor's Postscript

Wellness isn't a palace you arrive at. It's a very long stone path you keep walking down. This year, while I was editing *Firewalkers*, I went through a time of collapse. I was a ghost girl living in dream time. The whole time I kept thinking about Debra's story – resenting the world requiring anything of her except for getting out of bed. Or even for requiring getting out of bed.

I kept telling myself: *You have to walk through the fire to create the fire.* I said to myself, *I'm going to be like those people in the Firewalkers stories, and I'm going to look back and see that when I emerged I had something in my life that I didn't have before.* I kept thinking about people's stories. I kept hearing lines from the book in my head. And I kept reminding myself: *Someday I'm going to be glad I went through this.* Even though I couldn't really imagine that was true. It was like this little thread I was holding on to. I had to believe. But it was hard to believe.

You walk through the fire and you come out covered in ash and it feels surreal. When I think about how much *Firewalkers* changed my life, I wish there was a way to get this book into the hands of every person like me. Every person who doesn't have a thread to hang onto. If you read this book and it means something to you, please write and let us know. Please consider passing on this copy to someone else, or donating some copies to your local library or mental health center, or you can make a donation to our organization and we will give away books and work together to carry forward the message of hope. The mustard seed of hope.

Visit us at <u>**www.thefirebook.org**</u>.

*Please consider passing on
this copy to someone else.*

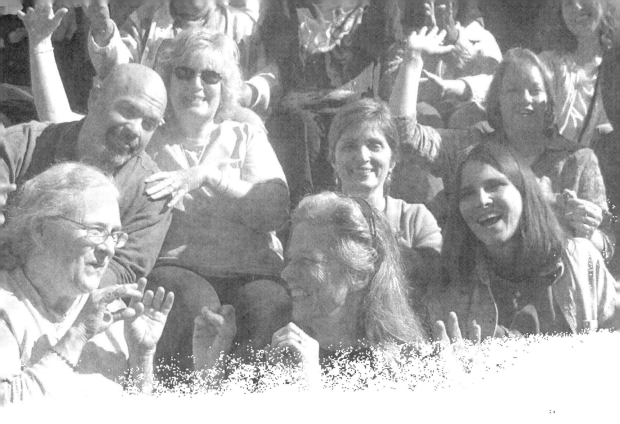

VOCAL is a nonprofit organization of people in mental health recovery. We are a community, support network, social change movement and self-help education program. VOCAL focuses on creating broad-scale social change, as well as change in the lives of individuals. We seek to transform the Virginia mental health system—and create alternatives to the system—by promoting mental health recovery, self-determination, and peer leadership.

As people who have personally experienced mental health crisis, we work to create programs that respect the inherent worth and dignity of all people, regardless of their current or past mental state, diagnosis, or use of medications. We value self-determination and the many important contributions of peer support and self-help.

Please consider making a tax-deductible contribution to support mental health recovery and disability rights. Visit www.vocalvirginia.org and find the "Donate" link.

Find out more about VOCAL at **www.vocalvirginia.org**, (434) 243-7878, *network@vocalvirginia.org*.

To order more copies of this book or find out more about *Firewalkers* please visit us at **www.thefirebook.org**. If you would like to write to someone in the *Firewalkers* book, please send your letter to *firewalk@ vocalvirginia.org*.

CPSIA information can be obtained at www.ICGtesting.com
Printed in the USA
BVOW060241120912

300228BV00003B/2/P